THE BATON SHOULD NOT FALL

Essential Read for a Young Medical Doctor
from a Renowned Cardiologist–Educator

B. Soma Raju
Arun Tiwari

Sakal Publications

Sakal Publications

THE BATON SHOULD NOT FALL

Sakal Media Pvt. Ltd.
595, Budhwar Peth,
Pune – 411002, India

www.sakalpublications.com
sakalprakashan@esakal.com

First Edition: October 2024

ISBN No.: 978-93-89834-92-5

Edited by: Anupama MA

Cover Design: Charumathy Murali

Typesetting: MAP Systems, Bengaluru

Printed in India by Sakal Media Pvt. Ltd.

An ideal of service permeates all our activities: service especially to the patient, as a fellow creature isolated on the island of his suffering, whom only you can restore to the mainland of health. For that purpose, you must know thoroughly not only the diseased but also the healthy.[1]

Felix Marti-Ibanez

In *To Be A Doctor*

1 Felix Marti-Ibanez, *To Be a Doctor, The Young Princes, The Race and the Runner*, New York: MD Publications, Inc., 1968.

Contents

Foreword ... 7
Introduction ... 9

Chapter 1 – Hippocrates ... 23
Chapter 2 – William Osler ... 37
Chapter 3 – Tinsley Harrison ... 55
Chapter 4 – Alexis Carrel ... 71
Chapter 5 – Eugene Stead ... 89
Chapter 6 – Edmund Pellegrino ... 107
Chapter 7 – The Lost Art of Healing ... 123
Chapter 8 – Practicing Right Medicine ... 141
Chapter 9 – Preserving the Passion ... 157
Chapter 10 – Health Systems Science ... 173

Epilogue ... 191
Acknowledgements ... 195
Index ... 197

Foreword

In "The Baton Should Not Fall: Essential Read for a Young Medical Doctor," Dr. B. Soma Raju, a distinguished Cardiologist Educator with a remarkable six-decade tenure, extends a bridge between the legacy of medical pioneers like William Osler and Tinsley Harrison to the aspiring doctors of today.

Through his extensive experience and unwavering dedication to cardiology, Dr Raju illuminates the paths paved by these giants of modern medical practice and provides practical applications of their wisdom, offering invaluable insights and timeless wisdom to the next generation of healers.

As readers embark on this enlightening journey through the corridors of medical history and innovation, they will witness the torch of medical excellence passed from the past to the present, ensuring that the essential principles and values these revered figures advocate remain steadfastly upheld in medicine.

"The Baton Should Not Fall" is not just a book but a guidebook for young doctors, a testament to the enduring legacy of those who have shaped the field. It is a powerful tool that inspires and empowers tomorrow's healers to carry the torch with passion, skill, and compassion, shaping their successful careers.

Dr. M. Srinivas, M.Ch.,
Professor of Pediatric Surgery & Director,
All India Institute of Medical Sciences, New Delhi

Introduction

When I completed 75 years on September 25, 2023, I asked myself, what next? As a Cardiologist, I did my DM from PGI, Chandigarh, in 1980. I have attended to close to a million patients in my OP clinic; I pioneered interventional cardiology in Andhra Pradesh in 1984, developed an indigenous coronary stent with legendary scientist Dr APJ Abdul Kalam in the mid-1990s and established the Care Foundation and Hospitals Network in 1997. I taught as a professor of cardiology at the Osmania Medical College and the Nizam's Institute of Medical College, and I held the dean's office at the latter. Of course, as some friends lamented, I did not create a medical college, but not a month passed when I did not take a class for the medical students who kept coming to me.

The idea for this book came to me from my friend and colleague, Prof Arun Tiwari, a missile scientist, and a pupil of Dr Kalam. He joined me in developing the stent and later co-founded Care Foundation. Prof Tiwari co-authored the legendary autobiography of Dr Kalam – Wings of Fire. Published in 1999, this book turned out to be a modern classic and, in its 70th reprint, sold more than 2.2 million copies, which is a record for any Indian book of this kind. His idea was that we write a biographical book about me, but I declined for two reasons. First, I was not sure if I would interpret the situations I went through correctly without confronting and even contradicting some luminaries of the medical profession, and second, much more important than what has happened is what should have happened but could not be. We felt that the best thing to leave behind as a legacy is the written words that would help those seeking guidance.

The history of the modern medical profession is a complex and multifaceted journey that has evolved over centuries in the Western world and has completed 100 years even in India. The history of medicine can be traced back to ancient times. Indian healers relied on a blend of empirical knowledge and mystical beliefs to treat illnesses. The basis was on harmonising the internal milieu, which was thought of as working as water, air, and fire – *kapha, vata, pitta.* Regulation of breathing and integration of body and mind is also emphasised as yoga. Even ancient Greeks believed in four humours. The transformation into a structured and scientific medical profession in Europe began in the late Middle Ages. It gained momentum through the Renaissance, eventually leading to the establishment of modern medical practices. Modern medicine arrived in India through the British, who ruled here for 90 years till 1947.

It is important to know that medical knowledge has always been intertwined with religious and philosophical doctrines. Monasteries served as centres for healing, and monks played a crucial role in preserving and transmitting ancient medical texts. The Renaissance in Europe marked a turning point in the history of medicine. During this period, there was a revival of interest in classical Greek and Roman texts, including works by Hippocrates and Galen. The printing press played a pivotal role in disseminating medical knowledge, making texts more accessible and facilitating the standardisation of medical education. The scientific revolution ushered in a new medical era in the 17th century. The work of scientists like William Harvey, who described blood circulation, and Andreas Vesalius, who revolutionised anatomical studies, laid the foundation for a more systematic and evidence-based approach to medicine. The concept of experimentation and observation became integral to medical practice.

The 18th and 19th centuries saw the formalisation of medical education and the establishment of medical schools. Medical societies and organisations were founded to regulate the profession and set standards for training and practice. The development of the microscope and advances in pathology contributed to a deeper understanding of diseases at the cellular level, leading to breakthroughs in diagnostics and treatment. The 19th century also witnessed the rise of medical specialisation, with physicians focusing on specific fields such as surgery, internal medicine, and obstetrics. The discovery of anaesthesia and the development of antiseptic techniques by figures like Joseph Lister revolutionised surgery, making it safer and more effective.

The turn of the 20th century brought about significant advancements in medical science. The identification of bacteria as the cause of infectious diseases, the development of vaccines, and the discovery of antibiotics marked milestones in preventive and curative medicine. Medical research and clinical trials became essential components of the profession, leading to the establishment of evidence-based medicine. In the mid-20th century, we witnessed the emergence of medical ethics and the formalisation of codes of conduct for healthcare professionals. The Nuremberg Code and the Declaration of Helsinki set ethical standards for medical research involving human subjects. Simultaneously, the development of healthcare systems and the expansion of public health initiatives aimed to improve the overall well-being of communities.

The latter part of the 20th century and the early 21st century saw rapid technological advancements in medicine. The introduction of medical imaging, the mapping of the human genome, and breakthroughs in biotechnology have transformed diagnostics and treatment modalities. Telemedicine has also emerged as a revolutionary concept, enabling remote patient care and consultation.

From here, my personal story gets entangled. Born the son of a farmer in the West Godavari district in the coastal Andhra region celebrated as the Rice Bowl of India, I got to study medicine by chance rather than design. I graduated from Guntur Medical College and even failed in my second year because of my philandering and passion for playing cricket. However, one chance discovery of William Osler's *Aequanimitas* in the college library where I sheltered myself one rainy afternoon changed my life, and I never looked back after that.

After practicing in government hospitals and private sector hospitals and spending time in some of the best hospitals in the United States and UK, I have experienced first-hand the challenges modern medical profession faces, such as ethical dilemmas, issues of access to healthcare, and the integration of artificial intelligence into medical practice. But one thing is obvious: despite these challenges, the medical profession's journey from its ancient roots to the present reflects a remarkable evolution marked by scientific inquiry, ethical considerations, and a commitment to improving the health and well-being of individuals and communities worldwide. There can be no better destiny for a human being than to be a medical doctor and care for needy patients. No profession in the world provides an opportunity, like medicine, to serve humanity. Dr Kalam used to call doctors second only to God in their work.

The history of Western medicine in India is a fascinating narrative that spans a little over one century, marked by interactions between indigenous healing practices and the introduction of Western medical knowledge. Here is a concise overview of the critical milestones in this historical journey: Before the arrival of Western medicine, India had a rich tradition of indigenous medical systems such as Ayurveda, Siddha, and Unani. These traditional systems were deeply rooted in the country's cultural and philosophical fabric and had been practised for centuries. During the colonial period, British physicians began introducing Western medical practices. The creation of the Medical College of Bengal in 1767 marked the formal introduction of Western medical education in India. Subsequently, medical colleges were set up in Madras (1835) and Bombay (1845).

When I grew up, no doctor was around, and people were used to managing with herbs. But there was a deep understanding of diet, and everything consumed was seen as 'hot' or 'cold', and balancing was embedded in common sense. Western medicine was confined to cities and urban areas, and even there, amongst the elderly, it was initially seen with scepticism, and people held on to their traditional healing practices, not out of compulsion but by choice. After gaining independence in 1947, India underwent significant changes in its healthcare system. The newly formed government recognised the need for a comprehensive healthcare approach blending Western and traditional medicine. In 1956, the government established the Medical Council of India to regulate medical education and practice.

In the post-independence era, India witnessed the growth of a robust healthcare infrastructure, including medical colleges, hospitals, and research institutions. The emphasis on preventive healthcare, vaccinations, and maternal and child health became integral parts of the healthcare system. The development of the indigenous pharmaceutical industry, pioneered in Andhra Pradesh by a gentleman of my area, Gokaraju Subba Raju, aka G.S. Raju, played a crucial role in people embracing Western medicine, and, of course, treatments became better with every season, as I may say. Over time, Western medicine gained acceptance, especially as it demonstrated its effectiveness in dealing with specific diseases and surgical interventions. But other challenges needed to be met. The country struggles with accessibility, affordability, and the urban-rural healthcare divide.

Numerous medical colleges and hospitals were set up nationwide, enhancing healthcare infrastructure and providing medical services to a larger population. These institutions became centres for medical education, research, and patient care. Established institutions such as the All India Institute of Medical Sciences

(AIIMS) in 1956 marked a significant step in advancing medical education and research in India. This was followed by the creation of the Postgraduate Institute in Chandigarh, which became a model institution and contributed to training medical professionals and setting high standards for healthcare in the country. While the public sector played a pivotal role, the private sector also started to contribute significantly to the hospital industry. The growth of private hospitals, especially in urban areas, introduced advanced medical technologies and specialised services. This shift began a dual healthcare system in India, with public and private sectors coexisting. Advancements in medical technology also played a crucial role in shaping the hospital industry. The introduction of modern diagnostic and treatment technologies, including imaging equipment, surgical techniques, and laboratory facilities, enhanced the quality of healthcare services.

At the time of writing this book, the government is playing a crucial role in expanding the hospital industry by investing in public-sector hospitals. Numerous medical colleges and hospitals are being set up nationwide, enhancing healthcare infrastructure and providing medical services to a larger population. These institutions have become centres for medical education, research, and patient care. However, the question about the standards of medical education remains to be addressed. As people of my generation know well, whether the standards of medical education in India have been diluted, is a complex and debated issue. There are no back-and-white answers and valid diverse perspectives and various factors contribute to the ongoing discussions.

Over the years, the number of medical colleges in India has significantly increased to meet the growing demand for healthcare professionals. While this expansion has improved accessibility to medical education, concerns have been raised about the quality of education and infrastructure in some newly established institutions. The Medical Council of India (MCI), the regulatory body for medical education, faced allegations of corruption and inefficiency. In 2019, the National Medical Commission (NMC) Act replaced the MCI with the National Medical Commission (NMC). The establishment of the NMC aimed to bring about reforms in medical education and enhance transparency. However, opinions differ on whether the new regulatory framework has effectively addressed the issues. There have been efforts to strengthen accreditation processes and quality assurance in medical education. Bodies like the National Board of Examination (NBE) and the National Accreditation Board for Hospitals and Healthcare Providers (NABH) assess and maintain the standards of medical education and healthcare services.

The rapid expansion of medical colleges has sometimes outpaced the development of infrastructure and faculty resources. This has led to concerns about the ability of some institutions to provide a high-quality learning environment. Faculty shortages, outdated facilities, and a lack of clinical exposure can affect the overall educational experience. The system of medical entrance examinations has changed, including the introduction of the National Eligibility cum Entrance Test (NEET) for admission to undergraduate and postgraduate medical courses. While standardised testing aims to ensure merit-based admissions, criticisms have been raised regarding the impact on candidates from diverse backgrounds and educational systems. Reports of corruption, malpractice, and fraud in medical education and entrance examinations have surfaced over the years, raising concerns about the ethical standards within the medical education system.

The government and regulatory bodies have addressed these concerns and implemented reforms. The introduction of competency-based medical education (CBME) and ongoing efforts to strengthen accreditation processes demonstrate a commitment to improving the quality of medical education. And I must not take sides or pass judgments. However, assessing standards in medical education requires a nuanced understanding of the complexities involved and ongoing initiatives to address the identified issues. Educating doctors involves a comprehensive approach that encompasses acquiring medical knowledge and technical skills and developing critical thinking, communication, empathy, and ethical values. The theme of this book is how to enhance medical education and produce better doctors.

Nothing is more important than an integrated curriculum. Designing and implementing integrated curricula that connect basic sciences with clinical practice and emphasise the relevance of theoretical knowledge to patient care is an SoS, if I may say so. Medical education fundamentally rests on clinical exposure. We must provide early and frequent clinical exposure to students, allowing them to observe and participate in patient care from the early stages of their education. Then there is what our teachers called 'bedside learning'. These are, in essence, methodologies that encourage students to actively engage with real-world medical cases, fostering critical thinking, teamwork, and problem-solving skills. Of course, I can see the arrival of integrated simulation-based training that allows students to practice clinical skills in a controlled environment, enhancing their proficiency and confidence before interacting with actual patients. Still, millions of patients in a country like India desperately need a doctor's presence and touch. Taking medical students not to the people is as severe as a sin.

However, the most crucial aspect of immediate remedy is fostering a culture of lifelong learning by promoting continuing medical education, encouraging participation in conferences, and facilitating access to up-to-date medical literature. Life cannot be lived online, and medical education without teachers and students dealing with patients 'together' is bogus and dangerous. Medical education ought to produce well-rounded, empathetic, and highly skilled doctors proficient in medical knowledge and technical skills and possess the interpersonal and ethical qualities necessary for excellent patient care. And this comes to the design of this book.

Studying the lives and contributions of great doctors can provide valuable insights and lessons for medical professionals at various stages of their careers. Great doctors often excel in clinical skills and diagnostic acumen. Studying their cases and approaches to challenging medical situations can enhance a doctor's clinical reasoning and decision-making abilities. Many renowned doctors are celebrated not only for their medical expertise but also for their dedication to patient-centred care. Learning about patient interactions, communication styles, and empathetic approaches can inspire doctors to prioritise their patients' well-being and experience. Great doctors are often characterised by their compassion and empathy. Reading about their experiences can encourage doctors to better understand patients' emotions, needs, and fears, fostering a more empathetic approach to healthcare.

Some great doctors have significantly contributed to public health by advocating for health policy changes, disease prevention, and community health initiatives. Doctors can learn about the impact of public health advocacy and consider ways to contribute to broader healthcare improvements. Many exceptional doctors have been pioneers in medical research and innovation. Exploring their contributions can inspire doctors to engage in research, stay informed about advancements in their field, and contribute to the evolution of medical knowledge and technology. Some doctors are recognised for their humanitarian efforts, providing medical care in underserved areas, participating in medical missions, or contributing to disaster relief. Learning about these experiences can encourage doctors to explore opportunities for humanitarian work and global health initiatives.

Great doctors often navigate complex ethical dilemmas with integrity and a commitment to patient welfare. Studying their ethical decision-making processes can help doctors develop a solid moral foundation and navigate challenging situations professionally. Many distinguished doctors exhibit strong leadership skills in clinical settings, research institutions, or healthcare organisations. Understanding their leadership styles and strategies can inspire doctors to cultivate practical leadership skills in their practice or healthcare settings.

A strong foundation of medical knowledge essentially demands the ability to stay updated with advancements in medicine, which are happening at a good pace. But what is perhaps most important is the ability to communicate clearly and be empathetic with patients, their families, and healthcare teams. Understanding and caring for patients' feelings and experiences helps build trust and rapport. It is also crucial to be meticulous in assessing the patient's condition before prescribing medications and providing treatment.

Maintaining high ethical standards and demonstrating respect, integrity, and responsibility in practice is becoming increasingly difficult. Even more challenging is collaborating effectively with other healthcare professionals to deliver the best patient care. The ability to handle stress and adapt to changing situations or challenges in the healthcare environment is the new hallmark of a successful doctor. All these qualities help medical doctors excel in their practice and positively impact their patients' lives.

Lastly, but most importantly, great doctors may have faced personal or professional challenges and setbacks. Reading about their resilience, perseverance, and ability to overcome obstacles can motivate doctors to navigate their challenges with determination and optimism. Great doctors often demonstrate a commitment to lifelong learning. Their pursuit of knowledge, engagement with medical literature, and participation in professional development activities can serve as a model for doctors to adopt a continuous learning mindset throughout their careers. In essence, exploring the lives and experiences of great doctors can provide a multifaceted source of inspiration, offering lessons on clinical excellence, patient-centred care, compassion, advocacy, innovation, ethical conduct, leadership, and resilience. This knowledge can contribute to doctors' professional and personal growth as they strive to deliver high-quality healthcare and make meaningful contributions to medicine. You are a good doctor already, why don't you become great?

Hyderabad
June 2024

Dr B. Soma Raju

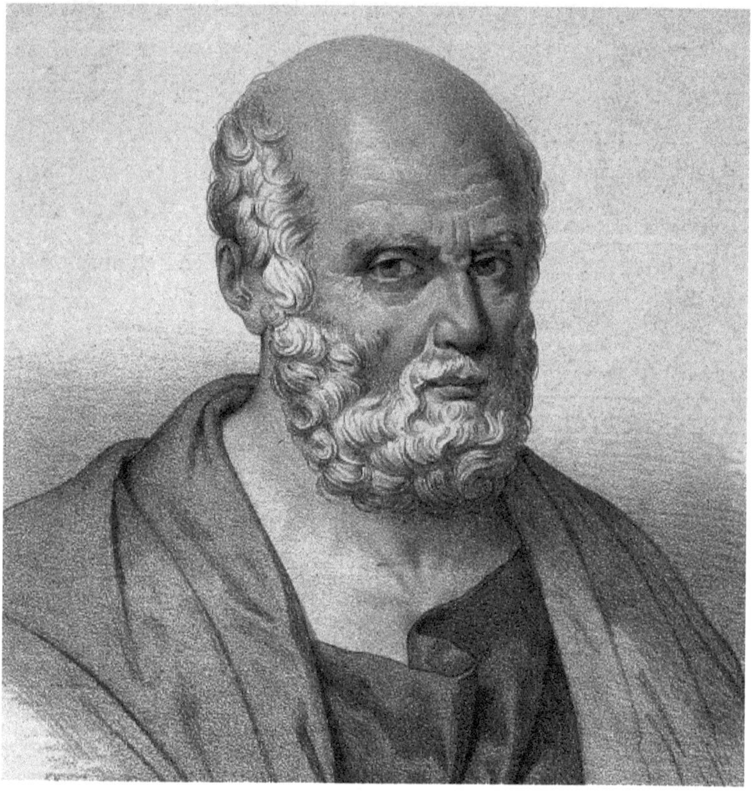

Chapter 1
Hippocrates

Hippocrates, often called the "Father of Medicine," is celebrated for his foundational contributions to medicine and influence on modern medical principles. While the appellate of a "Father" may be a simplification, it reflects Hippocrates's historical significance and contributions to establishing a rational, empirical, and ethical approach to medicine. His legacy is embedded in the foundations of modern medical principles, and his influence continues to be acknowledged and celebrated in the medical community.

Hippocrates lived between 460 and 370 BCE in ancient Greece. His teachings and practices represent a crucial turning point from superstition and mystical beliefs about human disease and death to a more systematic and rational approach to healthcare. In the ancient world, priests and magicians treated the sick in various ways, whimsical and weird. Gold, silver, mercury, and many strange things were used as medicines. Hippocrates was the first person in human history to write about medicine. Later, the collection of his and his disciples' writings, including numerous medical texts, case histories, and treatises, was compiled and called the "Hippocratic Corpus." They indeed form the foundation of medical knowledge.

Departing from the mystical and speculative approaches of his time, Hippocrates encouraged physicians to observe and document symptoms, the progression of diseases, and the effects of treatments - observational and empirical medical methods based on experience and a doctor's " guesstimate" without having every fact at his disposal - as they evolved from there. Patients go to senior doctors relying on their experience to diagnose and prescribe good treatment accurately. The Hippocratic Oath, said to have been told by Hippocrates, is translated into English here.

> I swear before my gods, my ancestors, my teachers, my fellow healers and apprentices, and by all the arts and knowledge I was privileged to learn that I will stand by these words:
>
> I will love those who taught me these arts as I love my parents, and I will offer my skills to the young with the same generosity they gave me. And I will never ask them for gold but demand that they stand by this covenant in return. I also swear that if I earn fame and wealth, I will share it with my masters and students.
>
> I will soothe the pain of anyone who needs my art, and if I don't know how I will seek the counsel of my teachers.
>
> I will offer those who suffer all my attention, my science and my love. Never will I betray them or risk their well-being to satisfy my vanity. I will not hurt my fellow or put a knife to his flesh if I don't know how or give him an herb to soothe his pain, even if he begs for it in anguish if it might take away his breath.

> I will never harm my suffering friend because life is sacred, from the tender fruit that he once was in his mother's womb to that first sigh he gave out between her legs when he opened his eyes to the world.
>
> I will try to understand his sorrows, but his secrets will never leave my ears. Under no circumstance will I use his body to advance my knowledge or my fame unless, in his last moment, he or his widow give me his corpse so that his death may help me understand how to soothe another's pain.
>
> I pray that the attention I give to those who put themselves in my hands is rewarded with happiness. And in honour of the knowledge I've received from my teachers, I swear to care for anyone who suffers, prince or slave.
>
> If I ever break this oath, let my gods take away my knowledge of this art and my health.
>
> Here speaks a citizen, a servant of people. May I be destroyed if I betray these words?[1]

A mix of stern civic ethics and inspired humanitarianism, the above text has endured to this day, not just under its literary merits but because it is the first definition of the medical profession, a written agreement and guideline for teachers, colleagues, and students of the healing arts as if a covenant of what to do and what not to do. This oath abides a doctor to *primum non nocere*, a Latin

---

1 https://www.bu.edu/arion/files/2010/03/Arenas_05Feb2010_Layout-3.pdf. Last accessed on March 11, 2024.

phrase that means "first, do no harm." The oath also signifies the importance of patient confidentiality and the recognition of the physician's responsibility to uphold ethical conduct. Little wonder that The Hippocratic Oath has profoundly influenced medical ethics throughout history.

The image of Hippocrates is often depicted holding a staff with a snake coiled around it—the Rod of Asclepius, the Greek god of healing and medicine. Hippocrates's legacy extends across various facets of medicine, ethics, and education. His holistic approach to patient care, emphasis on empirical observation, commitment to ethical conduct, and contributions to medical literature have shaped the foundations of modern medicine and continue to influence healthcare practices and principles today.

The system of medicine evolved after Hippocrates, but it remained overburdened with dogmas. Scholasticism, a bunch of words based on irrational faith, was a big part of early medical art. Words written by "scholars" controlled minds, and religion added its own beliefs. Even reasonable people thought that God was good and that all illnesses came from the devil. Interestingly, while the British Medical Association and World Health Organization correctly use the Rod of Asclepius in their logos, most of the hospitals use the staff of Hermes, with two snakes – in their logos, which is indeed the magic wand carried by Hermes, the messenger of the gods in Greek mythology. The rod with a snake best depicts the importance and hazards of the medical profession.

Life was considered natural, and disease supernatural. As late as the eighteenth century, the Scottish physician John Brown

(1735 - 1788) created a theory that regarded and treated disorders as caused by disturbance in the body's harmony. The Brunonian system of medicine, as it was called, had temporary success in America, Italy, and the German-speaking part of Europe. The extensive use of alcohol and opium brought it to disrepute soon, but the observation of Brown that perfect health in every aspect seldom happens to mortals became an axiom.

German philosopher von Schelling (1775 – 1854) regressed medicine into superstition. He believed disease was caused by a wide range of supernatural forces rather than problems functioning the body's systems. It was thought that a mind full of sin could turn a body's life from ordinary to pathological. People prayed and believed in religious dogmas to fix this. In a great travesty, medicine had returned to where it all began after several hundred years and would wait for the Industrial Revolution in the 18th century for a redux.

Several work-related diseases became more common as more industrial processes were automated. People who worked with phosphorous, usually in the match business, got lung disease, dermatitis, and "phossy jaw," a type of jaw necrosis. As cities increased, more people got diseases like typhus and cholera. As people moved from one part of the world to another, they brought diseases. Most notably yellow fever, with patients bleeding into the skin and cell death in the liver and kidneys was brought into Europe and America by slaves from Africa.

The biggest accomplishment of modern medicine is eliminating outdated ideas which stem from superstition and ignorance that date back hundreds of years, and replacing them with more scientific, humane, and often healing ways. It is astonishing how late, in its very long history of medicine, therapies of proven effectiveness were established. The progress made in basic science and the creation of epidemiological methods used to study causal connections are two of the most critical tools that made doctors learn about the causes and mechanisms of diseases.

Post-World War II, the number of hospitals, doctors, and researchers in the United States increased. From 1950 to 1970, the number of people working in medicine grow exponentially. Medicine has changed from a simple, natural, and personal field to a complicated, interdependent, and impersonal one. However, even though medicine was changing quickly, the framework and organisation of how services were provided didn't change much. Why should doctors promise the gods that they will keep the pact, even if it meant going against their best judgment? Dr Louis Lasagna, the academic dean of the School of Medicine at Tufts University in 1964, changed the Hippocratic Oath and aligned it with the times.

> I swear to fulfil, to the best of my ability and judgment, this covenant:
>
> I will respect the hard-won scientific gains of those physicians in whose steps I walk, and gladly share such knowledge as is mine with those who are to follow.
>
> I will apply, for the benefit of the sick, all measures [that] are required, avoiding those twin traps of overtreatment and therapeutic nihilism.

I will remember that there is art to medicine as well as science and that warmth, sympathy, and understanding may outweigh the surgeon's knife or the chemist's drug.

I will not be ashamed to say "I know not," nor will I fail to call in my colleagues when the skills of another are needed for a patient's recovery.

I will respect the privacy of my patients, for their problems are not disclosed to me that the world may know. Most especially must I tread with care in matters of life and death. If it is given me to save a life, all thanks. But it may also be within my power to take a life; this awesome responsibility must be faced with great humbleness and awareness of my own frailty. Above all, I must not play at God.

I will remember that I do not treat a fever chart, a cancerous growth, but a sick human being, whose illness may affect the person's family and economic stability. My responsibility includes these related problems if I am to care adequately for the sick.

I will prevent disease whenever I can, for prevention is preferable to cure.

I will remember that I remain a member of society, with special obligations to all my fellow human beings, those sound of mind and body as well as the infirm.

If I do not violate this oath, may I enjoy life and art, respected while I live and remembered with affection thereafter. May I

> always act so as to preserve the finest traditions of my calling and may I long experience the joy of healing those who seek my help.[2]

As I write this in 2024, sixty years later, the Oath still has some moral and societal meaning. It makes you think about moral qualities, talks about service and teamwork, and value learning, practice, wisdom, and knowledge. On the other hand, it doesn't fit with modern ideas about ethics, human rights, what society values, or scientific medicine. This is because the doctor and the relationship between the doctor and patient is no longer the only one responsible for safe health care. Some other factors have come up.

Now, diagnosis and treatment are more than just the job of doctors; biomedical engineers and technicians are also involved. Biotechnology, medical computing, and the new biosciences have made health care a broad-based delivery system. Using the Internet, people can learn a lot about their health, access care from many places, and decide what they need from their healthcare. They probably will need more than one doctor's care when they get sick. What used to be a direct relationship between a doctor and a patient - simple and stable – is now complicated.

Medicine, too, has changed. It happens more now in private spaces than in public ones, in more of a business world instead of a social one. Doctors meet patients in a clinic or visit bedside, but

---

2 https://www.pbs.org/wgbh/nova/doctors/oath_modern.html#:~:text=I%20swear%20to%20fulfill%2C%20to,those%20who%20are%20to%20follow. Last accessed on March 11, 2024.

the treatment is delivered in a complex organisational structure. Putting patients' needs first has become quite challenging. Patients might get hurt or harmed because of the complex web of human relationships within a wide range of technological and organisational structures that all work independently and are somewhat unpredictable. Hiding such errors makes them even more harmful.

In the early 1980s, the first reports of damage from health care were published in the United States. Since then, governments focused on healthcare safety, quality, and harmful events, and the medical profession responded wholeheartedly. In hospitals, incident reporting is now routinely used to identify medication errors, misidentification of patients, and operation theatre checklists. Much work has been done to reduce adverse incidents and improve the safety and quality of healthcare. However, a safer and more effective patient-centred healthcare system still needs to be found and reporting adverse events is a work in progress.

While human errors are inevitable, the healthcare system is also not free from mistakes. When hospital teams use root cause analysis to determine what went wrong, they usually find a series or a combination of several things that could have led to adverse results. For example, patients may be given the wrong medication they may be allergic to, a wrong dose, or scheduling test, a surgical procedure on the wrong side or the wrong part of the body, and even oversight of essential test results. Doctors and nurses should ask both the patients and their attendants extensive questions about their medical history, family history, treatments received and even make small talk. This kind of dialogue with the patients helps prevent many errors.

It is not doctoring alone; the knowledge and skills of many different health professionals make a difference. Health professionals must be technically skilled and able to speak clearly with their patients, their caretakers, and with each other so that patients can get the best care possible. A crucial part of knowing health care as a system is that different health professionals' ability to communicate quickly and efficiently affects patient care. I will return to this part, which discusses the need for health systems science, near the end of the book.

The medical field needs to work hard to keep the trust of patients and the public. The first codes of ethics made it clear to patients what they could expect from a doctor who follows the Hippocratic approach. There's no getting around the fact that patients are often hurt by their healthcare. Most of these problems aren't caused by doctors or trainees being careless or unethical but by gaps in understanding modern healthcare's context, changeability, and complexity.

A revised Hippocratic, published in the Journal of Medical Internet Research, reflects the 21st-century realities of medicine.

> I will respect the hard-won scientific gains of those physicians, researchers, and patients in whose steps I walk and gladly share such knowledge as is mine with those who are to follow.

> For the benefit of the healthy and the sick, I will apply all measures [that] are required, avoiding those twin traps of overtreatment and therapeutic nihilism.
>
> I will remember that there is an art to medicine as well as science, and that warmth, sympathy, and understanding may outweigh the surgeon's knife, the chemist's drug, or the programmer's algorithm.
>
> I will treat my patients in an equal-level partnership, and I will not be ashamed to say 'I know not,' nor will I fail to call in my colleagues when the skills of another are needed for a patient's recovery.
>
> I will respect the privacy of my patients and their data, for their problems are not disclosed to me that the world may know.
>
> I will remember that I do not treat a fever chart, a cancerous growth, a data point, or an algorithm's suggestion, but a human being.[3]

In the future, doctors will have to consider whether the medical-industrial complex will transform doctors as we know them and make doctors and workers of big businesses more accountable to their employers than their patients. They must deal with more flexible technological medicine that may take doctors even further

3 https://www.jmir.org/2022/9/e39177. Last accessed on March 11, 2024.

away from their patients' bedsides, affecting the relationship between patient and doctor.

The number of people moving into cities often exceeds the current healthcare system's capacity. Too many people in hospitals and clinics can prolong wait times and lower the level of care. Telemedicine, remote monitoring, and health information systems can enhance access to healthcare services and improve overall efficiency in urban healthcare delivery. Public health programmes, education, and lifestyle changes can help lower the number of people with chronic diseases in cities.

All these problems in medicine today impact the central relationship between the doctor and the patient in their unique ways. Hippocrates lives on in the hearts of doctors who think that the way medicine is changing now can change and strengthen the medical field. Doctors are determined to keep the unbreakable link between commitment and care in the world we live in now. To deal with these growing problems, the health industry needs to change with the times and focus on ways to keep diseases from happening.

How can doctors follow Hippocrates in their practice in modern times? It is a matter of capturing the philosopher's paramount concern for the patient's well-being by adhering to his espoused fundamental ethical guidelines and practices, with patient-centred care as its hallmark. A doctor must show genuine concern for the patient's well-being, listen actively, respect their feelings and perspectives, and consider their physical, emotional, social, and environmental factors when diagnosing and treating illnesses.

But perhaps the most important is the *primum non nocere* principle of non-maleficence—avoiding any harm to the patient in the treatment. I see a double whammy here. While superstition and magic remain even amongst the educated, the infusion of technology in medicine has further increased the possibility of harm to patients during treatment. Hippocrates remains relevant even in the 21st century. A doctor must avoid treatments or interventions that may harm the patient by weighing the potential benefits of treatment against the possible risks and side effects. A doctor must act in the patient's best interest by always prioritising the health and well-being of the patient in every decision and continuously improving the practice by staying updated with medical advancements to provide the best possible care.

Respecting a patient's privacy has assumed grave dimensions with camera-loaded mobile phones everywhere. Maintaining patient confidentiality, protecting their health information, and fostering trust by discerning and respecting patient privacy is hard and unavoidable. A doctor must be honest with patients about their diagnosis, treatment options, and prognosis while adhering to ethical guidelines set by medical boards and professional organisations. Fundamentally, patients are fully informed about their conditions, treatment options, and potential outcomes. By embodying these practices, modern doctors can honour the legacy of Hippocrates and maintain high ethical standards in their training, ensuring the best possible outcomes for their patients.

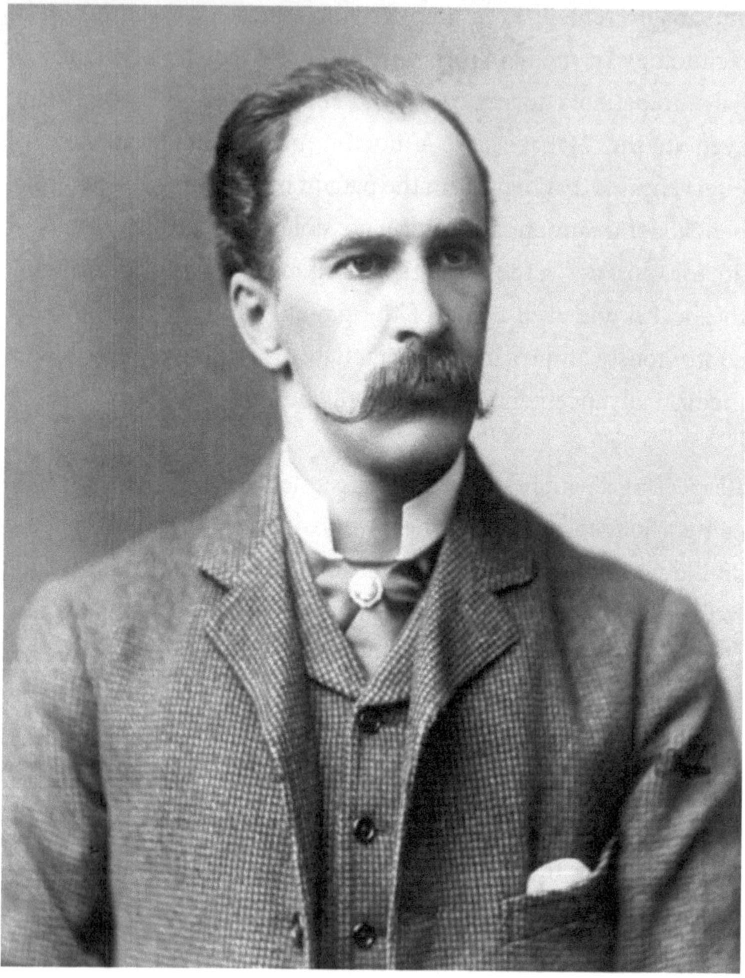

Chapter 2
William Osler

Sir William Osler (1849–1919), one of the founders who taught at Johns Hopkins School of Medicine, is known as the "father of modern medicine." He changed the way medical education was taught. I learned about him through his book *Aequanimitas,*[4] which I found in the library of Guntur Medical College. It was a collection of writings, starting with one of Dr Osler's lectures to newly graduated doctors at the Pennsylvania School of Medicine in 1889 as a farewell speech before moving to Johns Hopkins Hospital in Baltimore. I am citing four passages from this lecture here.

First, Dr Osler tells the young people in the room to "think about just two of the scores of things that can make or break your lives." The first is imperturbability, which means "calmness in a storm, clarity of judgment in times of great danger." He says this calm, poker-faced attitude is necessary to build trust in easily influenced or scared people. They expect their doctor not to be as anxious,

---

4 https://archive.org/details/aequanimitaswit04oslegoog. Last accessed on March 12, 2024.

agitated, and apprehensive as they are but to be confident, cooperative, and calm.

> In the first place, in the physician or surgeon, no quality takes rank with imperturbability, and I propose for a few minutes to direct your attention to this essential bodily virtue . . . Imperturbability means coolness and presence of mind under all circumstances, calmness amid storm, clearness of judgment in moments of grave peril, immobility, impassiveness, or, to use an old and expressive word, phlegm. It is the quality which is most appreciated by the laity, though often misunderstood by them, and the physician who has the misfortune to be without it, who betrays indecision and worry, and who shows that he is flustered and flurried in ordinary emergencies, loses rapidly the confidence of his patients.

Now, Dr Osler emphasises the need to be tolerant of people around you and not to react to provocations, which are galore in a hospital setting—sick patients, anxious attendants, harassed hospital employees, touts and paddlers, egoist bosses, and people of society smacking with their pride and entitlements.

> In the second place, there is a mental equivalent to this bodily endowment, which is as important in our pilgrimage as imperturbability . . . a calm equanimity is the desirable attitude . . . One of the first essentials in securing a good-natured equanimity is not to expect too much of the people amongst whom you dwell . . . Deal gently then with this deliciously credulous old human nature in which we work, and restrain your indignation . . . expect them, and do not be vexed.

Our needs define our expectations, and as doctors, where immense efforts are invested in becoming one, it is natural to have high expectations in life. If not me, who? Perhaps the most troublesome expectation is people helping you in your work and affection in your relationship. Dr Osler says that it is pre-decided that you will get disappointed and hurt. Adding from experience, this leads to the feeling of self-loathing as I may feel that it's my fault to expect from people. This creates a sense of dissatisfaction in my person and in the bonding I share. And lastly, it will make a conflict of interest, and in many cases, I may overthink my worth and allow people using me.

A doctor's life is a daily challenge. You don't even know which patients will meet you today with what problem and fate. Who more than doctors suffer this stress every day, their entire lives? It is natural for a doctor to see patients dying, and there is nothing much that can be done for it to be otherwise.

> It is sad to think that, for some of you, there is in-store disappointment, perhaps failure. You cannot hope, of course, to escape from the cares and anxieties incident to professional life. Stand up bravely, even against the worst . . . there is a struggle with defeat which some of you will have to bear, and it will be well for you in that day to have cultivated a cheerful equanimity. Remember, too, that sometimes "from our desolation only does the better life begin." Even with disaster ahead and ruin imminent, it is better to face them with a smile and with the head erect than to crouch at their approach. And, if the fight is for principle and justice, even when failure seems certain, where many have failed before,

> cling to your ideal . . . blow the challenge, and calmly await the conflict.

Dr Osler asks doctors to stick to their professional standards and ethics and be ready to fight any compromises. Finally, Dr Osler points to existence as a continuum. More than just doctors, we are also human beings who like everyone else must live and work in society and must leave sooner or later. Being grateful to our predecessors and having a sense of commitment to give and teach our juniors is an essential part of the medical profession, and it is no wonder it is called 'practice'.

> The past is always with us, never to be escaped; it alone is enduring; but, amidst the changes and chances which succeed one another so rapidly in this life, we are apt to live too much for the present and too much in the future. On such an occasion as the present, when the Alma Mater is in [the] festal array when we joy in her growing prosperity, it is good to hark back to the olden days and gratefully to recall the men whose labours in the past have made the present possible.

It took some time to understand the meaning of these passages and internalise the quality of staying calm and composed. Based on my own five decades of medical practice, I can say without hesitation that a good doctor must learn to be cool and present in mind under all circumstances. I must caution you here that some of my colleagues have interpreted equanimity as apathy—the absence of emotions—and others have practised it as measured or moderated emotions. Equanimity, in my opinion, comes from being accepting and not too quick to judge other people.

Dr Osler was instrumental in establishing teaching hospitals as centres for medical education. He believed that hospitals should serve as dynamic environments for learning, research, and patient care. His advocacy for the residency system, where newly graduated physicians receive advanced training in a specific medical speciality, contributed to the development of structured postgraduate medical education. He used every occasion in his illustrious career at the Johns Hopkins Hospital, considered the best teaching hospital in the world , to reflect on the virtues of student life and the formative experiences that shape aspiring physicians. He underscores the significance of cultivating a strong work ethic, perseverance, and a commitment to lifelong learning during the student years. Dr Osler demystified and defined the relationship between teachers and students in medicine. He advocated for a collaborative and mentorship-oriented approach, emphasising the role of teachers in inspiring and guiding the next generation of physicians.

In Osler's view, a medical doctor is both a caregiver and a man of science. He encourages physicians to balance clinical skills and commit to advancing medical knowledge through scientific inquiry. He also stresses on following the Oslerian ideals of calmness, empathy, and a deep commitment to the art and science of medicine. Osler's legacy endures in the principles and values he advocated for in medical practice and education. Osler's addresses have profoundly impacted medical education, promoting the importance of bedside teaching, clinical experience, and a humanistic approach to patient care. His teachings have influenced generations of medical educators and practitioners. I tried to emulate Dr Osler in my clinical training and bedside teaching as a medical student and later as a teacher. Osler advocated for a shift from a solely didactic approach to medical education, promoting hands-on experience with patients at the bedside. Osler believed exposure to real clinical cases was essential for developing practical clinical skills and diagnostic acumen.

Dr William Osler's relevance was paramount in integrating basic sciences and clinical medicine, and his approach laid the groundwork for a more comprehensive and holistic medical education curriculum. Dr Osler is even more important today when technology has increased in every aspect of healthcare delivery. Medical students must understand the scientific principles and technology underlying clinical practice. I watched in horror how the Medical Council of India destroyed medical education before the organisation was dismantled, which was a little too late. The restoration remains a work in progress, and I am duty-bound to record the Five-fold shift, which I consider for good medical education here.

1. Patient-Centered Education: This paradigm shift towards patient-centred medical education places the patient at the forefront of the learning experience. It should emphasise the importance of understanding and addressing patients' needs, preferences, and values to improve the quality of healthcare delivery. Effective communication is a cornerstone of patient-centered education. Students learn to communicate empathetically and respectfully with patients and their families. This includes active listening, providing information in understandable

language, and addressing patients' concerns. A Medical student must be provided opportunities to engage in real-world experiences, such as clinical rotations and community-based care, to enhance their understanding of patient-centred principles in actual healthcare settings.

2. Integrating Basic and Clinical Sciences to provide a holistic understanding of medical principles and their practical applications in patient care. The idea is to combine the foundational knowledge of basic sciences with clinical applications, creating a seamless and interconnected learning experience for medical students. The goal is to present medical knowledge cohesively and interconnectedly by integrating basic sciences principles, such as anatomy, physiology, biochemistry, and pathology, with clinical disciplines like internal medicine, surgery, and paediatrics. This would incorporate problem-based learning (PBL) methodologies to present students with clinical cases and guide them to explore relevant basic science concepts to solve clinical problems. PBL fosters critical thinking and the application of knowledge in clinical contexts.

3. Return to Teaching at the Bedside: About a quarter of clinical teaching occurred at the bedside seventy-five years ago. Today, that number is only about ten percent. Doctors' lack of exposure to an essential part of training during their undergraduate years is partly to blame because more and more patients are discussing it. Students

can connect directly with patients, watch for clinical signs, and improve their communication and examination skills by teaching them at the bedside. This helps them feel more comfortable talking to and examining actual patients with the help of a more experienced practitioner. Teaching at the bedside also opens people's minds to the real world of health, which actors can't do. Getting a full background from a patient sensitively and correctly can take some time.

4. Lifelong learning echo system: Role modelling is essential in professional development. It is a set of activities demonstrating the knowledge, skill, attitude, and ethical behaviour students should acquire. A mentorship and role-modelling culture can be achieved by fostering programs that connect students with experienced faculty members and practitioners, promoting positive role-modelling and professional development. It is necessary to cultivate an eco-system of continuous quality improvement, regularly evaluating the effectiveness of the educational program and making enhancements based on feedback and outcomes data. Role modelling is one of the best approaches for cultivating professionalism in medical students. A word of caution I must add here. A mentor can show a good example and teach best practices. In contrast, a role model can offer positive and negative examples, and it will be up to you to understand the difference and learn only good.

5. Effective Use of Technology: Leverage technology for educational purposes, including virtual learning

resources, telemedicine, and electronic health records, to prepare students for the evolving healthcare landscape. Using technology in medical education can help students learn basic information more quickly, make better decisions, see things in multiple ways, coordinate their skills better, prepare for rare or essential events, learn how to work as a team, and improve their physical skills. All of these goals can be met with different tools. The job of medical educators is to make good use of these new tools so that learning is more collaborative, personalised, and empowering. Anyone can learn anything from anyone in our world at any time. It is obsolete and even considered obnoxious, for patients to tell about who they are, bring old records, and repeat tests every time they visit a hospital.

By incorporating these five shifts, medical education programs can prepare students to meet modern healthcare's complex challenges, promoting clinical competence and the values and attitudes essential for providing compassionate and patient-centred care.

In the rest of this chapter, I share ten of Dr Osler's quotes from his extensive writings. I must confess that these quotes have often inspired and guided me in my personal and professional life as a doctor, teacher, and in my public life.

1. The personal ideals:
   I have had three personal ideals: One, is to do the day's work well and not to bother about tomorrow. You may say that is not a satisfactory ideal. It is, and there is not

one which the student can carry with him into practice with greater effect. To it more than anything else I owe whatever success I have had — to this power of settling down to the day's work and trying to do it well to the best of my ability, and letting the future take care of itself. The second ideal has been to act the Golden Rule, as far as in me lay, toward my professional brethren and toward the patients committed to my care. And the third has been to cultivate such a measure of equanimity as would enable me to bear success with humility, the affection of my friends without pride, and to be ready when the day of sorrow and grief came, to meet it with the courage befitting a man. What the future has in store for me, I cannot tell — you cannot tell. Nor do I care much, so long as I carry with me, as I shall, the memory of the past you have given me. Nothing can take that away.[5]

2. Caution against professional arrogance in the medical profession:
   Perhaps no sin so easily besets us as a sense of self-satisfied superiority to others. It cannot always be called pride, that master sin, but more often it is an attitude of mind which either leads to bigotry and prejudice or to such a vaunting conceit in the truth of one's own beliefs and positions, that there is no room for tolerance of ways and thoughts which are not as ours are.[6]

5 Silverman Mark E., Murray, Jock T, and Brayan Charles S., The Quotable Osler, Philadelphia: American College of Physicians, 2008, p 3.

6 Ibid. p. 9.

3. The master-word in medicine is work.

   I propose to tell you the secret of life as I have seen the game played and as I have tried to play it myself... Though a little one, the master word looms large in meaning. It is the open sesame to every portal, the great equaliser in the world, the true philosopher's stone, which transmutes all the base metal of humanity into gold. The stupid man among you will make bright, the bright man brilliant, and the, brilliant student steady. With the magic word in your heart all things are possible, and without it all study is vanity and vexation. The miracles of life are with it; the blind see by touch, the deaf hear with eyes, the dumb speak with fingers. To the youth it brings hope, to the middle-aged confidence, to the aged repose. True balm of hurt minds, in its presence, the heart of the sorrowful is lightened and consoled. It is directly responsible for all advances in medicine during the past twenty-five centuries . . . And the master-word is Work, a little one, as I have said, but fraught with momentous sequences if you can but write it on the tablets of your hearts and bind it upon your foreheads.[7]

4. The best part of a doctor's work is influence and comfort.

   Often, the best part of your work will have nothing to do with potions and powders or with the exercise of an influence of the strong upon the weak, of the righteous upon the wicked, the wise upon the foolish. To you, as the trusted family counsellor, the father will come with his

7 Ibid. p. 33.

anxieties, the mother with her hidden grief, the daughter with her trials, and the son with his follies. Fully one-third of the work you do will be entered in other books than yours. Courage and cheerfulness will not only carry you over the rough places of life, but will enable you to bring comfort and help to the weak-hearted, and will console you in the sad hours when, like Uncle Toby [a compassionate character], you have 'to whistle that you may not weep'.[8]

5. The Value of Experience is to see wisely.
   The important thing is not to make the lesson of each case tell on your education. The value of experience is not in seeing much, but in seeing wisely. Experience in the true sense of the term does not come to all with years, or with increasing opportunities. Growth in the acquisition of facts is not necessarily associated with development. Many grow through life mentally as the crystal, by simple accretion, and at fifty posse, to vary the figure, the unicellular mental blastoderm with which they started. [9]

6. Wisdom comes from relating facts and experience.
   The facts are looked at in connexion with similar ones, their relation to others is studied, and the experience of the recorder is compared with that of others who have worked upon the question. Insensibly, year by year, a man finds that there has been in his mental protoplasm not only

8 Ibid. p. 47.
9 Ibid. p. 198.

growth by assimilation but actual development, bringing fuller powers of observation, additional capabilities of mental nutrition, and that increased breadth of view which is of the very essence of wisdom.[10]

7. Good teachers teach the best information and create new knowledge.
   The function of the teacher is to teach and to propagate the best that is known and taught in the world. To teach the current knowledge of the subject, he professes—sifting, analysing, assorting, and laying down principles. To propagate, i.e., to multiply, facts on which to base principles—experimenting, searching, testing. The best that is known and taught in the world—nothing less can satisfy a teacher worthy of the name.[11]

8. Truth grows and evolves.
   Like a living organism, Truth grows, and its gradual evolution may be traced from the tiny germ to the mature product. Never springing, Minerva-like, to full stature at once. The truth may suffer all the hazards incident to generation and gestation. Much of the history is a record of the mishaps of truths which have struggled to the birth, only to die or else to wither in premature decay. Or the germ may be dormant for centuries, awaiting the fullness of time.[12]

---

10 Ibid. p. 199.
11 Ibid. p. 231.
12 Ibid. p. 269.

9. We will always be sad.
   Sorrows and griefs are companions sure sooner or later to join us on our pilgrimage, and we have become perhaps more sensitive to them, and perhaps less amenable to the old-time remedies of the physicians of the soul; but the pains and woes of the body, to which we doctors minister, are decreasing at an extraordinary rate, and in a way that makes one fairly gasp in hopeful anticipation.[13]

10. Selfless service to others is the best way to fight depression.
    Let us bury the sorrows of yesterday in the work of today. A little tincture of Saturn may be allowed in our hearts, but never in our faces. Sorrow and sadness must come to each one—it is our lot. We can best oppose any tendency to melancholy by an active life of unselfish devotion to others.[14]

What makes an ideal doctor of the 21st Century? What would Dr William Osler say to a young medical graduate of 2024?

The ideal physician in the modern world possesses medical expertise, interpersonal skills, adaptability, and ethical values. A perfect physician understands and connects with patients emotionally, demonstrating empathy and compassion, leading to a supportive and trusting doctor-patient relationship. The healthcare landscape continually evolves with new technologies, treatments, and delivery models. Doctors need to be tech-savvy, adaptable, open to change, and willing to embrace new approaches

13 Ibid. p. 280.
14 Ibid. p. 280.

for the benefit of their patients. Embracing and leveraging technology, such as electronic health records, telemedicine, and diagnostic tools, is essential for providing modern, efficient, and high-quality healthcare and is fundamental, not even an option.

However, maintaining the highest ethical standards is of paramount importance. Nothing is hidden in the modern connected world. Physicians must prioritise patient welfare, confidentiality, and informed consent and act with integrity in all professional interactions. Even your thoughts are deciphered by artificial intelligence through your phones and computers. Only doctors practising in patients' best interests, including their rights to quality care, undertaking informed decision-making, and mobilising their access to necessary resources, will flourish hereafter. Dr William Osler may even say that life can't be wellness since it is not virtual. He would advocate realism in all aspects of living, including medicine.

Dr Osler emphasised the importance of bedside teaching and the human side of medicine, advocating for a more compassionate and personalised approach to patient care. Osler's legacy shaped medical education and practice throughout the twentieth century, inspiring generations of healthcare professionals, myself included, to prioritise the well-being of their patients. In the last two or three decades, bedside teaching in hospitals has undoubtedly faced challenges, with the increasing demands on healthcare providers and the emphasis on technology-driven medicine.

Medical professionals and educators of my era still recognise the value of bedside teaching in providing a holistic and hands-on learning experience for students. Efforts must be made to revive and preserve this art by incorporating it into medical school curricula and continuing education programs. By emphasising the importance of direct patient interaction and observation, bedside teaching helps trainees develop essential clinical skills, empathy, and critical thinking abilities. Senior physicians can take up honourary roles to impart bedside teaching to willing students. Over time, bedside teaching has evolved into a valuable and irreplaceable component of medical education and must be preserved.

The human side of medicine, including empathy, compassion, and patient-centred care, has faced challenges in the modern healthcare system. With the advancement of technology, increased patient volume, and administrative burdens, healthcare providers may sometimes need help to prioritise the human connection with their patients. And that help is non-existent. There is a growing recognition within the medical community of the importance of maintaining the human side of medicine.

Efforts must be made to promote patient-centred care, improve communication between healthcare providers—doctors and nurses—and patients, and emphasise empathy and compassion in medical education. Initiatives such as narrative medicine, cultural competence training, and patient advocacy programs are helping to reemphasise the importance of the human element in healthcare.

While systemic challenges can make it difficult for providers to prioritise the human side of medicine, many healthcare professionals continue to strive to maintain a patient-centred approach and a focus on the individual needs of those under their care. By acknowledging these challenges and actively working to address them, the human side of medicine can be preserved and strengthened in the face of modern healthcare demands. Senior physicians must show this by, for example, seeing patients in charitable hospitals even for a few hours and maintaining the sacred fire so it does not extinguish.

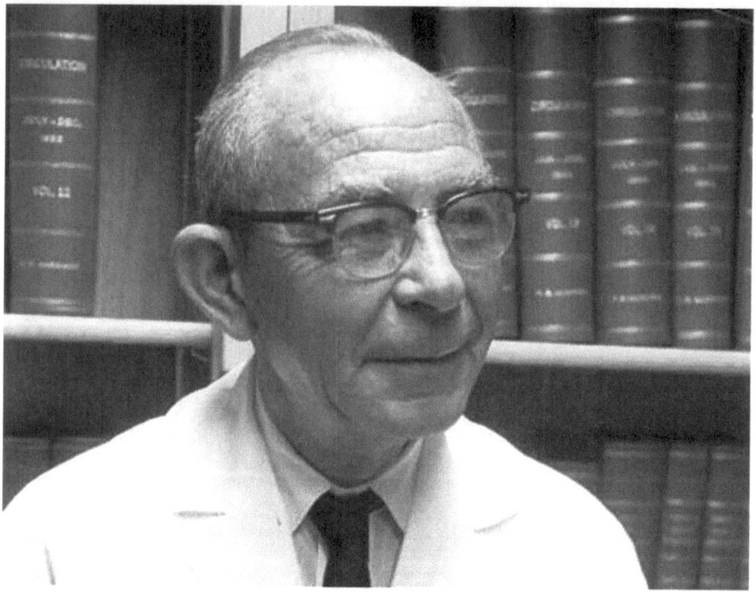

Chapter 3
Tinsley Harrison

Tinsley Harrison (1900–1978) was born in an ancestry of doctors. His father, William Groce Harrison, was a sixth-generation doctor who worked briefly with Dr William Osler. Dr Harrison was celebrated as a master of cardiac auscultation. He possessed a keen ear for detecting subtle heart sounds and murmurs and made precise diagnoses of various cardiac conditions by listening through his stethoscope. I was so fascinated when I read about him as a medical student that I convinced my patients in Guntur Medical College Hospital to allow me to hear their heart sounds for extended periods —a few times, even if it was an hour. Auscultation, considered the most crucial part of a heart clinical examination for a long time, is quickly becoming a lost art.

As a child, we look up to and respect older people. You can pick someone who has done great things or lives their life in a way you want—having someone to look up to can help you stay motivated and meet your goals. As a doctor, cardiologist, and educationalist, I modelled myself on Dr Harrison. Through his textbook, "Harrison's Principles of Internal Medicine," he remained my guide. I found it as a scripture—every time I read it, I learned something new and gained insights. Using the words of Shakespeare, Dr Harrison asked a doctor to be interested in both the wise and the stupid, the proud and the humble, the strong hero and the whining rogue. He must never discriminate and choose in his care for people but serve all who arrive.

The general availability of more complex and pricey high-tech diagnostic and therapeutic methods, especially Doppler echocardiography, has made it easy for many young doctors to refrain from indulging in cardiac auscultation beyond a point. But I have to tell the young doctors that cutting-edge high technology is not a replacement for a strong background in clinical cardiology, which includes heart auscultation. The stethoscope is still a valuable and inexpensive medical tool as long as it is used correctly. A good doctor can quickly and accurately diagnose heart problems with few or no extra tests. Each person does not need every test.

When I was working in PGI, Chandigarh, a healthy 23-year-old Sikh farmer was brought to the hospital with a lung embolism that could kill him. Even after a complete medical study that included a coagulation workup, we still didn't know what caused it. We put him on anticoagulation medicine to save his life, but I was not too fond of it because the young man would no longer be able to do the things he wanted, like pulling weights, swimming, and running. I developed a friendship with the young man, making him agree to let me listen to his heart in various positions and when he moved his limb. After some time, I noticed he missed a beat when his arm moved behind his back. The sound went away when he turned his head but returned when he looked forward. It didn't take me long to figure out that the man had thoracic outlet syndrome, which is when the blood vessels under the collarbone get squished, not letting blood flow to the arm. The problem was fixed with a minor surgery, and the young man was taken off anticoagulation treatment. He had no trouble going back to work in his field.

It is not only auscultation, but overall, the trend of physical examination is fading out. Of course, there are time constraints, but that has always been the case. I have seen a hundred patients daily in my OP and never skipped a physical examination. How long ago was the last time you gave a patient a complete physical exam? Is the physical test a lost art in the medical field today? I'm afraid so. But I am sure that it should not be allowed. Getting clinical signs was the most crucial part of learning medicine in medical school. The medical students were there to listen to the symptoms and get a complete background. It was my favourite thing to go to the intensive care units to hear the early diastolic murmurs in the aorta area and the pan systolic murmur in the mitral area. Later, looking for the third heart sound (S3), a rare extra heart sound that occurs soon after the usual two "lub-dub" heart sounds (S1 and S2), became my passion. This sound represents a transition from rapid to slow ventricular filling in early diastole and is a hallmark of heart failure.

The idea of clinical medicine has been turned on its head by modern medicine and technology. Molecular biology techniques and other lab investigation methods are more accurate. Imaging methods have also changed a lot, making it possible to diagnose complex problems immediately. No wonder young doctors spend time at the computer in their practice. The clinical medicine of the past is outmoded because of all the new technology, but it must be preserved. However, technology is not the problem; it is how people use it. Technology is helpful because it shows us parts of the patient's body that we can't see. However, it can't tell us about a sore spot in the belly, a raised jugular venous pulse, or how the patient felt that morning.

In my college days, the grand rounds were essential to bedside clinical activities. During these rounds, the medical history and current ailments of every patient was talked about in detail with the whole staff and resident body present. Today's rounds are done before a computer screen, looking at a picture or lab tests. Everyone but the patient seems to be part of these rounds. Many patients in Accidents or Emergency (A&E) or the wards miss a diagnosis because their physical check isn't done right. The patient's medical history and a physical check are essential to making a correct diagnosis. Lab tests and imaging studies, on the other hand, serve to support these findings. Combining the intelligent use of technology with the personal touch that is so important to the sacred bond between a doctor and a patient is the only way to move forward. Technology and a physical check will improve diagnostic accuracy, cut unnecessary tests, and help doctors get closer to their patients and "feel" their pain.

Dr Harrison was known for his exceptional diagnostic skills in cardiology. His thorough physical examinations of patients allowed him to gather comprehensive information about cardiac function and identify abnormalities. Dr Harrison was an early advocate and adopter of echocardiography. He became head of the Department of Medicine at the University of Alabama School of Medicine in Birmingham in 1948. This leadership role provided him a platform to influence medical education at institutional and national levels. He played a pivotal role in shaping medical education methodologies and curriculum development. His commitment to excellence in education set a standard that resonated across the medical community.

It is here that Dr Harrison wrote the legendary textbook *Principles of Internal Medicine* (PIM). Initially published in 1950, it has undergone multiple editions, each reflecting the evolving landscape of medical knowledge. Celebrated for its depth, clarity, and relevance, it is an indispensable resource for medical students, residents, and practitioners worldwide. While Dr Tinsley Harrison was the primary author, the textbook has involved multiple contributors and editors. Dr Harrison writes in the first and last paragraphs of his introduction to PIM in 1950.

> No greater opportunity or obligation can fall the lot of a human being than to be a physician. In the care of suffering he needs technical skill, scientific knowledge, and human understanding. He who uses these with courage, humility, and wisdom will provide a unique service to his fellow man and will build an enduring edifice of character within himself. The physician should ask of his destiny no more than this and he should be content with no less.
>
> Tact, sympathy, and understanding are expected of the physician, for the patient is no mere collection of symptoms,

> signs, disordered functions, damaged organs, and disturbed emotions. The patient is human, fearful, and hopeful, seeking relief, help and reassurance. To the physician, as to the anthropologist, nothing human is strange or repulsive. The misanthrope may become a smart diagnostician of organic disease, but can scarcely hope to succeed as a physician. The true physician has a Shakespearean breadth of interest in the wise and the foolish, the proud and the humble, the stoic hero and the whining rogue. The physician cares for people.[15]

The collaboration of experts in various medical specialities ensures the inclusion of diverse perspectives and the incorporation of the latest medical advancements. The content is designed to bridge the gap between theoretical knowledge and its practical application in clinical settings. Real-world case studies and examples help readers understand how medical principles are applied in patient care. Besides physical examination, "Harrison's Principles" also emphasises evidence-based medicine, encouraging readers to critically evaluate research literature and apply scientific principles to clinical decision-making.

Ideally, integrating evidence-based practices reflects the evolving nature of medical knowledge. However, as I observed, it has been taken a little too far, to the extent that a physical examination is considered a wasteful exercise. In this chapter, I discuss how evidence-based medicine (EBM) has become the usual way to make clinical decisions in my practice. You must

15 Piiman, James A., *Tinsley R. Harrison: Teacher of Medicine,* Montogomery: New South Books, 2015, p. XXVI-VI

combine your clinical experience with the best external clinical evidence from systematic studies to practise evidence-based medicines. However, this has become an end in itself. Test results based on scientific evidence have replaced methods like clinical epidemiology, systematic search, and meta-analysis for evaluating and combining outside evidence. Other methods like cost analysis and modelling were also mostly thrown out. While "Harrison's Principles" are very different from EBM, they are becoming increasingly accepted as the best way to make medical practice and policy decisions as medical insurance grows.

Many doctors in clinical practice are averse to EBM, as do people who study philosophy, health sociology, and implementation science. Even EBM researchers who used to back the movement are calling for a "renaissance," especially when it comes to the parts of EBM that involve making decisions with patients and using evidence-based expert judgment. The main worry is the harmful effects on healthcare policy, service, and funding. EBM has made life more like a medical problem by making up new diseases for vague complaints and using "quality markers" to push drugs and medical devices to a broad audience.

Rather than leading to a diagnosis, many test results lead to another set of tests, and the cascade continues, searching for evidence of some anomaly rather than the ailment. Young doctors must know this debate, for it is loaded with the consequences of the future of medicine. Here, I talk about four ways of thinking: how EBM came to be, its main ideas and factors, why this movement overgrew and was so well received, a "restricted" view of EBM, and how it can be used to create standard methods for developing practice guidelines; and the problems the EBM movement is currently facing in the areas of systems thinking and implementation sciences.

Three things gave rise to the evidence-based medicine movement. One, hospitals in the US went from places where sick people were housed to prestigious places where medical care is based on scientific principles. Second, medical education was changed; teaching hospitals sprung up, and clinical epidemiology was created. Along with hospital changes, healthcare services were becoming more consistent through guidelines. This was closely linked to the American Medical Association's efforts to become the leading medical accreditation group. Standardisation included regulating the medical field to ensure surgeons had the proper training, creating procedure standards in hospitals to reduce variation and boost quality, and adding the patient record file for the first time to let hospital managers keep an eye on what the doctors were doing. And third, professional autonomy grew as new scientific information and technologies emerged, along with standards and guidelines. However, as the new millennium began, too many standards and rules led to a loss of clinical autonomy.

Dr David Sackett at Canada's McMaster University created a "problem-based learning" programme in 1968 that combined the study of basic sciences, clinical epidemiology, and clinical medicine by using real-life problems as the basis for the lessons. Using what we learned from clinical statistics to improve clinical practice was a very new idea. In medical practice, terms like "levels of evidence" and "grading study designs" came into use and were used to grade treatment suggestions, ranging from "use the intervention" (Level A) to "do not use the intervention" (Level E). When computers came along, they made electronic records possible. Knowledge management, which used to be something only a few pros could do, became more open to everyone as computers got faster. After some time, The Cochrane Collaboration was formed as a group that carefully searched, reviewed, and compiled the vast body of research literature so that it could be easily used by doctors during patient consultations.

I don't know how it helped the clinical practice, but some new disciplines, such as health economics and outcomes management, were born. I must mention my amazement upon seeing the doctor-patient relationship becoming a profession-population issue leading to "business forecasting" and "growth rates" in the "healthcare industry". The three EBM approaches focused on the "specific" to reach measurable goals, continuously evaluating performance against clear goals, outputs, and standards, and allocating resources based on effectiveness criteria to make doctors' work more visible through oversight and control. These approaches have, ironically, led to pricing structures, disease-related groups, and lowering the costs of both operating rooms and operating room cabins.

Even more interesting was the idea behind the creation of Outcomes Management (OM), which used quality improvement principles to make it easier for doctors to be independent and in charge of their clinical practice. OM is based on four central ideas: 1) Appropriateness, which is based on standards and guidelines 2) Routing outcome assessment, which looks at how well patients are doing and how long they live, as well as disease-specific clinical outcomes at the right time points 3) Data mining to collect vast amounts of clinical and outcome data 4) Dissemination and impact analysis to look at the part of the database that is most relevant to each.

Like EBM, OM tried to give doctors the power to make better clinical decisions with the help of new tools. While OM was celebrated as returning the power of decision-making managers and auditors to clinicians, effectively, it ended the "old way" of "only" practising subjective medicine based on gut feelings, clinical experience, and pathophysiological reasoning. Instead, it replaced that with an objective method based on "scientific" evidence. They wanted evidence to be a significant factor, but they also strongly disagreed with the idea that experts with "authoritative opinions" should make clinical decisions. It was a new form of colonisation, funded by Big Pharma, as Europeans had come to Asia for trading and went to Africa to civilise it.

In hindsight, evidence-based medicine was different from the work of medical doctors. It was a big game rolled out by big money. I remember that the first paper on EBM to be published in the Journal of the American Medical Association (JAMA) was written by an EBM Working Group that kept their names private. It was made into an official agreement paper and backed up immediately by solid evidence. The EBM Working Group used words more like a political platform to call for significant changes in how medicine is done, which led to the creation of an "enterprise of scientific objectivity." Soon, the British Medical

Journal became a strong supporter of Europe. What seemed like overnight, evidence-based practice guidelines became the standard for government agencies and professional groups, and they are at the heart of modern scientific thought. Unfortunately, the scientific community didn't adopt EBM based on evidence but on expert knowledge. Is this different from the kind of method that EBM was meant to replace?

In 1995, *The Lancet* took a critical position on EBM. An anonymous editorial lauded the use of the best available evidence in practice but deplored attempts to make medicine an evidence-based field in and of itself. The opinion has been divided since then. There are doubts about the hierarchy of evidence for focusing only on internal validity and ignoring the vital issue of external validity or how those results can be used in other situations. An over-simplified approach to 'the clinical care of patients' was not what Hippocrates, Dr William Osler and Dr Tinsley Harrison had promoted.

Let me share an old phenomenon called the Matthew Effect with my young readers. It comes from a Biblical phrase (Matthew 25:29, RSV) - *For to everyone who has will more be given, and he will have abundance; but from him who has not, even what he has will be taken away.* It is used in the modern world to raise the credibility of a viewpoint by making celebrities state it. You can see film stars and sports champions promoting fashion and health products. In science, it is done by organising excessive cross-citation amongst its proponents. This power is exercised to set future research, practice, and policy agendas. Those who cite and celebrate specific ideas are given grants, invited for conference presentations, and even financed to hold positions in professional societies. In a few years, some of the 'commoners' turned into minor celebrities; what if their wise colleagues consider them jumping frogs in a well? I am not making my resistance to EBM an excuse for my oblivion in the research publications later in my career, for that is a different story. Still, at least in India, most celebrated clinicians shunned EBM.

It's important to remember that scientific knowledge is split into three main areas: finding, confirmation, and application. You can use more than what you learn in one area in the other two. The value-neutrality principle that leads to discovery and confirmation must be explained in more detail and complicated during the implementation phase. It means that the scientist removes scientific facts from fundamental beliefs about right and wrong as a means to an end. Means-end inferences and abduction are used in EBM guideline development without an adequate formalisation of their contribution to the construction of the guideline recommendations. Sadly, the philosophy of science ideas needed to support EBM's foundations has not been thoroughly researched.

Two-pronged validity is the most essential thing in discovery and confirmation. The study methodology ensures that there is a low risk of bias, which is called "internal validity." The results are also "externally valid" because they can be used in the real world and with this patient. Internal validity and outward validity are opposite to each other. External validity should be emphasised and strengthened if the end goal of EBM is to improve the health of real people in real situations. External validity means a treatment will work in controlled situations in the real world. Internal validity means that a treatment works in controlled conditions. Even though EBM's methods for grading clinical guidelines are organised and trustworthy, they often put too much emphasis on internal validity and are not "fit for purpose." A more fundamental question would be whether randomised controlled studies can be used to test or achieve real-world results. No, is my answer.

Most likely, EBM grew too quickly to fully embrace its original ideas based on evidence, expert knowledge, and patients' preferences. EBM worked well in the short term, mostly in single-disease conditions that could be treated easily. However, this method only works well in today's epidemiological setting, which is marked by chronicity and multiple morbidities in complicated health systems. In particular, EBM needs to pay more attention to the importance of social factors in health and the local context.

As a general rule, evidence depends on the situation. Both global and local evidence must be brought together to make valuable suggestions for treatment decisions. Local proof includes things like the nature of needs, the patient's values, the costs to both the patient and the system, and the resources available in the system. This local proof must be combined with "expert knowledge," which is not the same as "expert opinion" and should be given a higher value. "Expert knowledge" refers to the unspoken information that experts have that helps them understand how things work in a particular area. "Colloquial evidence" is always a part of making guidelines.

Artificial intelligence (AI) may lead to better evidence for clinical decision-making when defining "expert knowledge" in the study of research data. Substantial progress in smart tech, data science, and machine learning has started to change evidence-based medicine, giving us a compelling look into the future of "deep" medicine. The COVID-19 pandemic showed some problems with how clinical trials are usually run. Still, it also led to some good changes, such as new trial designs and a move towards a more patient-centred and easy-to-understand system. Fighting the coronavirus has led to massive progress in many fields, including genomics, immunology, proteomics, metabolomics, gut microbiomes, epigenetics, and virology. Big data science, computational biology, and artificial intelligence (AI) have sped up these improvements. Also, the rise of CRISPR–Cas9 technologies has created a lot of exciting new possibilities in personalised medicine.

Even with these improvements, they are not being quickly brought from the lab to the bedside in most areas of medicine, and clinical study is still behind. Millions of people still live with chronic diseases, and they cost society a lot of money in terms of loss of productivity and expenditure on life-long medication. However, the study is challenging because most data is stored in separate files. Because doctors are so specialised, there are now silos both within and between specialities. Each big disease area works on its own. Can machine learning, deep neural networks, and multimodal biological AI be used to change this? Does AI improve clinical research, drug finding, image interpretation, workflow, electronic health records, and public health in the long run? There are no definite answers, but "the physician should always ask of his destiny no more than this, and he should be content with no less, " so declared Dr Harrison.

Dr Harrison's dedication to medical education and passion for advancing the field of internal medicine have had a lasting impact on generations of healthcare professionals through his textbook. The book's 21st edition, published in 2022, is in two volumes. The editors of this edition include modern legends Dr Anthony Fauci (b. 1940), Dr Dennis Kasper (b.1943), Dr Stephen Hauser (1949), Dr Dan L Longo (b. 1949), Dr Joseph Loscalzo (b. 1951), and Dr J. Larry Jameson (b. 1952). In chapter 199 on Chapter 199: Common Viral Respiratory Infections, the SARS-CoV-2 virus, its clinical manifestations, management, and public health implications are included. Incidentally, Dr Anthony Fauci has played a crucial role during the COVID-19 pandemic as the Director of the National Institute of Allergy and Infectious Diseases (NIAID) in the United States.

Harrison's Principles of Internal Medicine remains the most trusted resource in a world influenced by endless sources of medical information. The latest edition includes new chapters on cutting-edge medical topics, such as immune checkpoint inhibitors, advances in precision medicine, and genetic therapies. Most importantly, online access is offered to supplemental materials, including videos, case studies, and self-assessment tools to support learning and clinical practice. Like a beacon of knowledge and excellence, it is unparalleled in any other discipline in accuracy and utility.

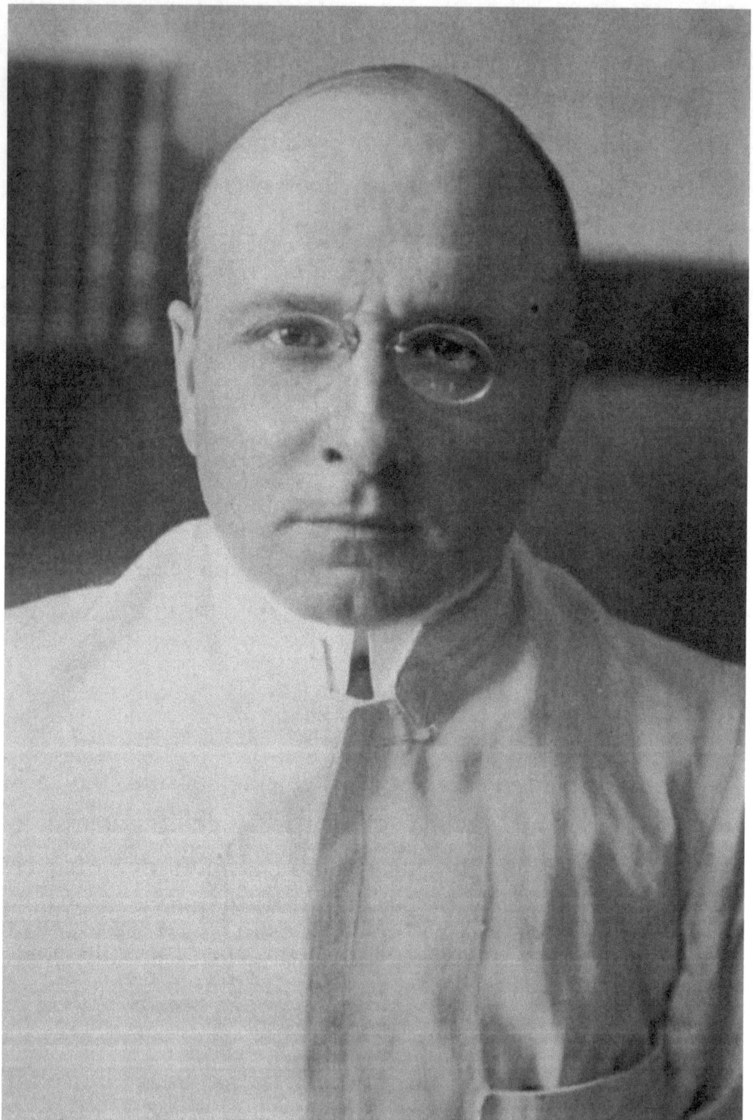

Chapter 4
Alexis Carrel

Each profession has one person who stands out as a great teacher, leader, or thinker. These things were true of Alexis Carrel (1873–1944), who worked in heart surgery. Marie Joseph Auguste, later shortened to Alexis Carrel, was a French scientist and surgeon who did most of his work in science in the United States. The Nobel Prize in Physiology or Medicine was given to Dr Carrel in 1912 for his work on vascular suturing methods and organ transplantation. The fact that current cardiovascular surgeons still use the vascular suturing techniques Dr Carrel first developed shows how great he was.

Dr Carrel not only developed innovative techniques for suturing blood vessels, which significantly advanced the field of vascular surgery, but his methods were also crucial for successful surgeries involving blood vessel repair and transplantation. Carrel's pioneering research in tissue culture laid the foundation for modern cell biology and biomedical research. He developed techniques for maintaining cells in culture outside the body, enabling researchers to study cellular behaviour and diseases in controlled laboratory settings.

Dr Carrel delves into the complexities of human physiology, discussing various bodily systems and their functions. He explores the intricacies of human biology, highlighting the wonders of the human body. Dr Carrel's research laid the groundwork for future advancements in organ transplantation. Although he did not directly perform organ transplants, his work on tissue culture and vascular techniques paved the way for later breakthroughs. His contributions continue to inspire researchers in various fields of medicine and biology.

Dr Carrel was also known for his philosophical and ethical reflections on science, medicine, and spirituality. I learned about Dr Alexis Carrel through his book *Man, The Unknown*, which explores the mysteries of human life, the potential of humanity, and the ethical implications of scientific progress. I read it during my stay in Chandigarh where I was first admitted for my super speciality in endocrinology. However, after a few months, I realised that endocrinology was not my calling and decided that it was not something I wanted to specialise in.

When I read *Man, The Unknown, it opened* new horizons for me. Based on new findings in biology, physics, and medicine, the book tried to give a complete picture of what is known and unknown about the human body and life. In hindsight, if Dr William Osler's *Aequanimitas* inspired me to become a doctor, Dr Carrel's *Man, The Unknown,* motivated me to become a cardiologist. Without hesitation, I decided to forgo one year of studying endocrinology and secured a DM seat in cardiology.

What I found unique in *Man, the Unknown* was how Dr Carrel saw the phenomena of life in their bewildering complexity and observed practically every form of human activity. The circumstances of Dr Carrel's life have led him to cross the path of philosophers, artists, poets, and scientists. And also of geniuses, heroes, and saints. At the same time, he has studied the hidden mechanisms which, in the depth of the tissues and the immensity of the brain, are the substratum of organic and mental phenomena.

Lourdes is a famous shrine to the Virgin Mary in southern France. The Catholic Church widely publicised the miraculous healing to people who prayed to Mary there. In 1903, Dr Carrel visited the shrine and encountered a very ill girl of 17. She was almost dead. It was likely that she had tuberculosis peritonitis, which is an inflammation of the peritoneum, which is the thin tissue that lines the inside of the belly and covers most of the organs there. Her abdomen was grossly distended by solid masses, her ribs protruded sharply, her legs were swollen, her heart rate and respiration rate were increased, and she had a high fever.

Members of her family had died of the same disease, and she was at Lourdes as a last resort. When the holy water was sprinkled upon the girl, Alexis Carrel saw her belly flat, and her heart rate and respiration turned normal. Within an hour, she seemed perfectly well and cured. Carrel thought he might be dreaming. He could not scientifically explain what he had seen. He wrote:

> Certain facts observed in Lourdes cannot be accounted for by any of the laws of wound healing and tissue regeneration. In the course of a miraculous cure, the rate of tissue construction greatly exceeds that which has ever been observed in the healing of a wound under optimal conditions. There is also a constant relation between the occurrence of this phenomenon

and the state of the prayer of the patient or someone near him. This fact cannot be accounted for.[16]

As a well-known doctor, his observations made headlines throughout France, with unfortunate results for Carrel. The clergy attacked him for being sceptical, and the medical community attacked him for being gullible. The two-pronged criticism made Carrel migrate to Canada. He aimlessly spent many months in different places in North America before he arrived in Chicago in September 1904.

At the beginning of the 20th century, it was believed that connecting arteries and veins was impossible. At the University of Chicago, between November 1904 and August 1906, Dr Alexis Carrel, assisted by Dr Charles C. Guthrie (1880 –1963), wrote several papers about connecting arteries and veins. They perfected a technique of inner coating closure by making three guide sutures on the outer wall. It was called triangulation anastomosis, a term for connecting tubular structures such as blood vessels or loops of the intestine. This would later win him the Nobel Prize at 39, the youngest scientist to receive the Nobel Prize in medicine.

Excellence attracts excellence. Harvey Cushing, the 'Father of neurosurgery' (1869–1939), asked Carrel to join him at the Johns Hopkins Hospital in April 1905. Dr Simon Flexner (1863–1946), a pathologist who was recently named head of New York City's brand-new Rockefeller Institute, was there. Flexner liked it so

---

16 Malinin T, *Surgery and Life, The Extraordinary Career of Alexis Carrel,* New York: Harcourt Brace Janovich, 1979.

much that he asked Carrel to join him there. Carrel shifted to New York in September 1905. Carrel's laboratory became a new meeting point for some of the outstanding people of that time.

William Welch (1850 –1934), physician, pathologist, bacteriologist and the first dean of the Johns Hopkins School of Medicine; William Halstead (1852 –1922), surgeon and an early champion of newly discovered anaesthetics; Karl Landsteiner (1868 –1943) immunologist, who distinguished the main blood groups in 1900 and would later win the Nobel Prize in 1930; and Rudolph Matas (1860 –1957), whom the "Father of Modern Medicine" William Osler (1849 - 1919) called the "Father of Vascular Surgery," were frequent visitors to Alexis Carrel's laboratory. Albert Einstein (1879 –1955) would drop in to discuss the supernatural with him while Alexis Carrel continued his work.

Alexis Carrel continued his journey to Lourdes every August for a long time. In 1910, he met Anne-Marie, who would become his wife. While I am not an atheist, religion never inspired me. Reading Dr Carrel's reflections on the spiritual dimensions of human life and the moral responsibilities of individuals and societies, I started spending some quiet time in contemplation. I understood the power of asking for guidance and support from a higher power.

> Prayer is a force as real as terrestrial gravity. As a physician, I have seen men, after all other therapy had failed, lifted out of disease and melancholy by the serene effort of prayer. Only in prayer do we achieve that complete and harmonious assembly

> of body, mind and spirit which gives the frail human reed its unshakable strength.[17]

Alexis Carrel stands out because of his transcendence of the narrow boundaries that define Medicine. He could see the shortcomings of humanity's way of life, especially the bad and harmful effects of progress and development. Dr Carrel explored the consequences of technological advancement and industrialisation on human values and societal well-being. *Man, the Unknown*, was perhaps his response to the sad situation of the world, not because of any natural calamity but the making of greed and power-mongering.

> Moral sense is almost completely ignored by modern society. We have, in fact, suppressed its manifestations. All are imbued with irresponsibility. Those who discern good and evil, who are industrious and provident, remain poor and are looked upon as morons. The woman who has several children, who devotes herself to their education, instead of to her own career, is considered weak-minded. If a man saves a little money for his wife and the education of his children, this money is stolen from him by enterprising financiers. Or taken by the government and distributed to those who have been reduced to want by their own improvidence and the shortsightedness of manufacturers, bankers, and economists. Artists and men of science supply the community with beauty, health, and wealth. They live and die in poverty. Robbers enjoy prosperity in peace. Gangsters are protected by politicians and respected

17 https://roerichsmuseum.website.yandexcloud.net/RD/RD-132.pdf (p. 22). Last accessed on March 13, 2024.

> by judges. They are the heroes whom children admire at the cinema and imitate in their games. A rich man has every right. He may discard his aging wife, abandon his old mother to penury, rob those who have entrusted their money to him, without losing the consideration of his friends. ...Ministers have rationalized religion. They have destroyed its mystical basis. But they do not succeed in attracting modern men. In their half-empty churches they vainly preach a weak morality. They are content with the part of policemen, helping in the interest of the wealthy to preserve the framework of present society. Or, like politicians, they flatter the appetites of the crowd.[18]

Carrel's criticism was not taken lightly by the forces running the world, including the medical establishment. No wonder Carrel is not celebrated in a manner befitting the magnitude of his contributions. I felt the strong influence of Alexis Carrel in various stages of my life. No human being can be fitted in a straight jacket of any profession, and medicine is no exception. A doctor remains a human being first, and his fears and concerns outside medicine play a part in his life. As depicted in a brilliant 1966 Hollywood film, there are three very different sides to the man and his work, which can be divided into the good, the bad, and the ugly.

Alexis Carrel was 21 years old and had already completed his medical degree when, in 1894, the president of the French Republic,

18 https://nige.files.wordpress.com/2011/02/alexis-carrel-man-the-unknown-1935.pdf (p. 124). Last accessed on March 13, 2024.

Sudi Carnot, was assassinated. Carnot had been stabbed in the abdomen and had survived long enough to reach the hospital, where a surgical incision into the abdominal cavity was made. It was found that the portal vein - a blood vessel that carries blood from the gastrointestinal tract, gallbladder, pancreas, and spleen to the liver -had been deeply cut. As surgeons had no means at their disposal for treating arterial and venous injuries other than by tying a ligature tightly around, the president bled to death. Carrel was convinced that the torn vein could have been repaired by itself. He spent the next five years experimenting on animals with fine needles and threads obtained from embroiderers. Eventually, he perfected arteri-venous anastomoses between dogs' carotid arteries and jugular veins. Carrel's early work with arterial suturing laid the foundations for today's surgical principles.

In his Nobel laureate lecture in 1912, Carrel described the complications of vascular suturing, namely stenosis, haemorrhage, and thrombosis, and how they could be avoided. He detailed the necessity of absolute asepsis and the need to handle vessels gently to prevent trauma and subsequent thrombosis. He described the importance of keeping the vessels' walls moist and flushing away foreign tissue or coagulated blood from the joining site.

> In operations on blood vessels certain general rules must be followed . . . [for] eliminating the complications which are especially liable to occur after vascular sutures, namely, stenosis, haemorrhage, and thrombosis. A rigid asepsis is essential. Sutures of blood-vessels must never be performed in infected wounds . . . It is possible that a slight non-

> suppurative infection, which does not prevent the union of tissues "per primam intentionem", may yet be sufficient to cause thrombosis . . . The desiccation of the endothelium may also lead to the formation of a thrombus. Therefore, during the operation the wall of the vessels must be humidified with Ringer's solution or be covered with Vaseline. The presence of coagulated blood, of fibrin ferment, or of foreign tissues or tissue juices on the intima can determine the production of a thrombus . . . Stenosis is very liable to occur at the point of anastomosis, therefore the suture must be performed while the wall is under tension. The tension can easily be obtained by traction on retaining stitches properly located . . . When these general rules are observed the operation can be safely performed.[19]

Having perfected the technique of suturing vessels, Dr Carrel experimented with the transplantation of arterial segments, which he harvested and preserved in cold storage. He was also able to transplant organs, including the kidneys and hearts of dogs successfully, and he even successfully transplanted the hind limb of a dog. Despite perfecting these surgical techniques, he was acutely aware of the problems of applying these techniques on humans. In 1908, the newborn baby of an influential New York doctor, Dr Lambart, was bleeding to the extent that death was inevitable. Dr Lambart convinced Carrel to carry out a procedure where his radial artery was connected to the popliteal vein of his infant daughter. The infant survived to adulthood.

---

19 https://www.nobelprize.org/prizes/medicine/1912/carrel/lecture/. Last accessed on March 13, 2024.

> Carrel reluctantly agreed and anastomosed the left radial artery of the father (the left arm was used because it was uncertain whether Dr Lambert would lose his hand, and the right-handed Adrian did not want to lose his good hand if he was to lose one to the popliteal vein of the infant using his triangulation technique. The baby became pink, stopped haemorrhaging, and was saved. So, incidentally, was Dr Lambart's hand. Thus, a leading vivisectionist had performed an operation, learned through vivisection, to save the life of an infant.[20]

Dr Carrel served in the French army during World War I. He knew that fighting in the trenches in the farmlands of rural France caused an unacceptably high number of illnesses and deaths from gas gangrene that spread from even minor cuts. He worked in a hospital on the front line at Compiegne with an English chemist, Henry Dakin. Together, they developed a wound management technique involving installing a sodium hypochlorite solution known as Dakin's solution. More important than using this local antiseptic in the pre-antibiotic era was Carrel's recognition of the importance of thorough and repetitive debridement of wounds and the need to remove all foreign material and devitalised tissue.

His colleagues considered Carrel's working methods to be unconventional. His laboratory was painted black to reduce glare from natural sunlight, and he and his staff wore black robes and caps. To maintain sterility, he actively discouraged visitors.

20 Walker, L.G., Carrel's direct transfusion of a 5-day-old infant. *SurgGynObst* 1973; 173:494-497.

It was interpreted as mysticism and scorned as eccentricity. The American Capitalists did not like his open criticism of greed, and though his scientific work could be addressed, his philosophical views were disdained.

> Modern civilization seems to be incapable of producing people endowed with imagination, intelligence, and courage. In practically every country there is a decrease in the intellectual and moral caliber of those who carry the responsibility of public affairs. The financial, industrial, and commercial organizations have reached a gigantic size. They are influenced not only by the conditions of the country where they are established, but also by the state of the neighbouring countries and of the entire world. In all nations, economic and social conditions undergo extremely rapid changes. Nearly everywhere the existing form of government is again under discussion. The great democracies find themselves face to face with formidable problems--problems concerning their very existence and demanding an immediate solution. And we realize that, despite the immense hopes which humanity has placed in modern civilization, such a civilization has failed in developing men of sufficient intelligence and audacity to guide it along the dangerous road on which it is stumbling. Human beings have not grown so rapidly as the institutions sprung from their brains. It is chiefly the intellectual and moral deficiencies of the political leaders, and their ignorance, which endanger modern nations.[21]

21 https://nige.files.wordpress.com/2011/02/alexis-carrel-man-the-unknown-1935.pdf (p. 22) Last accessed on March 13, 2024.

Influential critics were soon to point out that while expressing his views on spirituality while reinforcing his belief in the Darwinian principle of 'survival of the fittest', Dr Carrel did not include minority groups and was exclusively white. Dr Carrel even went on to offer a humane and economical solution. Rather than build more extensive and more comfortable prisons, he suggested they should be "disposed of" using "proper gases."[22] The controversy generated by the book almost certainly led to his forced retirement from the Rockefeller Institute and his return to France. There, he had the support of the French Vichy government and was successful in having them support the establishment of a 'foundation for the study of man' in 1942. This was to improve the world's population by scientific nutrition and public hygiene. It was also undoubtedly used to promote and perhaps promote action on his views of eugenics.

The institution was, of course, closed following the liberation of France in 1944, and it seems likely that Carrel would have faced arrest and be charged of being a 'Nazi supporter' after the war had he not died in 1944. Because Dr Carrel was famous, everything he said and did was closely examined. It could be argued that Carrel himself did no evil; he merely sympathised with and expressed views held by others who went on to carry them out in what was one of the most appalling chapters of European history. In 1991, when an ultra-right-wing party used Carrel's work to argue against the admission of immigrants to France, which they said would lead to the 'pollution' of the population, Carrel's name was removed from a small street near the Eifel Tower.

22 Ibid., p. 250.

I liked Dr Carrel and suggested that every doctor read his work to absorb his belief in humanity's immense potential to transcend its limitations and achieve greatness. Throughout the book, Carrel emphasises the ethical responsibilities of scientists and intellectuals. He warns against the misuse of scientific knowledge for destructive purposes and advocates for the ethical use of technology for the betterment of humanity. Overall, *Man, The Unknown* offers a profound exploration of human nature, spirituality, and the ethical dimensions of scientific progress. It challenges readers to reflect on the meaning of life, the pursuit of knowledge, and the responsibilities inherent in being human.

> The precision of any concept whatsoever depends upon that of the operations by which it is acquired. If man is defined as a being composed of matter and consciousness, such a proposition is meaningless. For the relations between consciousness and bodily matter have not, so far, been brought into the experimental field. But an operational definition is given of man when we consider him as an organism capable of manifesting physicochemical, physiological, and psychological activities. In biology, as in physics, the concepts which will always remain real, and must be the basis of science, are linked to certain methods of observation. For example, our present idea of the cells of the cerebral cortex, their pyramidal body, their dendritic processes, and their smooth axon, results from the techniques invented by Ramon Y Cajal. This is an operational concept. Such a concept will change only when new and more perfect techniques will be discovered. But to say that cerebral cells are the seat of mental

> processes is a worthless affirmation, for there is no possibility of observing the presence of mental processes in the body of cerebral cells. Operational concepts are the only solid foundation upon which we can build. From the immense fund of knowledge we possess about ourselves, we must select the data corresponding to what exists not only in our mind, but also in nature.[23]

Dr APJ Abdul Kalam publicly called *Man, The Unknown* amongst the great books that inspired him. We both saw in Dr Alexis Carrel a zeal that scientists have, significant ethical responsibilities beyond their pursuit of knowledge and advancement of science. Scientists should prioritise promoting human welfare and well-being in their research endeavours. This includes addressing societal challenges, improving public health, and advancing knowledge that can benefit humanity. When, in 1992, Dr Kalam took over as the Director General of the Defence Research & Development Organization (DRDO), he consulted me to start a Civilian Spinoff program utilising defence technology to provide affordable medical devices and consumables, mostly imported, to needy people at affordable prices through indigenous development. The celebrated *Kalam-Raju Stent* was a product of that initiative.

However, the most remarkable outcome was the innovation of floor reaction orthoses to support polio-affected lower limbs. Polio is a highly transmittable disease caused by a virus. It penetrates the nervous system and can cause complete paralysis in a matter of hours. The virus spreads primarily by the faecal-oral route or, even through contaminated water or food, though

23 Ibid., p. 30-31.

less frequently, and multiplies in the intestine. One in every 200 infections causes irreversible paralysis in the legs. Polio typically affects children under the age of five, and they live with this crippling disability for life.

My colleague, Dr B. N. Prasad, an Orthopedic Surgeon, literally forced Dr Kalam to see some such children when he came to see me in the hospital when we were discussing how to make stents indigenously. Seeing the plight of these children, mostly in their teen years, Dr Kalam was deeply moved and could not speak for a while. Dr Prasad suggested that we create lightweight support for their legs, which can transfer the body weight from the knee to the sole; these children can stand and even walk with a stick. This idea gave birth to Floor Reaction Orthosis (FRO), which is made of advanced composite material used to make missile nose cones. In an ultra-lightweight design, the FRO provides knee stability during walking. Later, some children fitted with FRO could even ride bicycles. Dr Kalam later said that as a scientist who worked for the betterment of society, it was his moral obligation to offer his expertise and support.

Polio is an incurable disease, but it can be effectively prevented through vaccination. When administered multiple times, the polio vaccination can provide lifelong immunity. And it eventually happened. India was declared polio-free in March 2014. To maintain the country's polio-free status, polio vaccination is part of mandatory immunisation in India. Inactivated Polio Vaccine (IPV) has also been introduced to further boost the population's immunity as additional protection against polio. Vaccination to international travellers to and from eight other countries and continuous vaccination at the international borders of India are being carried out throughout the year to mitigate the risk of importation.

Overall, Carrel's perspective underscores the idea that doctors have a moral obligation to consider the broader societal implications of their work and use their expertise to better humanity. By embracing their ethical responsibilities and joining hands with other scientists outside the medical fraternity, they can contribute to creating a more just, sustainable, and equitable world. Dr Carrell's famous observation that man exists midway between an atom and a star on a magnitude scale inspires me to think big but never miss the minute details.

Dr Carrel's legacy in medicine is significant and enduring. He pioneered the field of tissue culture, developing techniques to keep organs and tissues alive outside the body. His research in organ culture contributed to understanding cell biology and metabolism and paved the way for advancements in regenerative medicine and biomedical research. There is great promise for treating cardiovascular diseases by harnessing the body's natural ability to repair and regenerate damaged heart tissue. Functional heart tissue created in the laboratory using a combination of cells, biomaterials, and growth factors can be used for transplantation or to develop more effective drug screening platforms.

Regenerative medicine in cardiology is a rapidly evolving field with the potential to revolutionise the treatment of cardiovascular diseases. What interventional cardiology did in the 1980s will be repeated by regenerative cardiology in the 2030s. Gene therapy techniques will repair damaged heart tissue and promote cardiac regeneration by delivering genes to the heart that can stimulate tissue repair, enhance blood vessel growth, or improve heart function. Biomaterials and scaffolds will create supportive structures to guide heart tissue regeneration. These materials will also help deliver cells or growth factors to the damaged area and provide a framework for tissue regeneration. Induced pluripotent stem cells (iPSCs) are reprogrammable to differentiate heart muscle cells and hold promise for personalised regenerative therapies in cardiology.

As cell-based therapies continue to show promise in preclinical and clinical studies, the role of cardiologists in administering and overseeing these advanced treatments is likely to expand. The emergence of cell therapy in cardiology represents an exciting frontier in cardiovascular medicine, and Cardiologists will be mandated to collaborate closely with researchers, cell biologists, and other specialists to develop regenerative therapies tailored to individual patient's needs, ultimately aiming to enhance heart function, quality of life, and outcomes for individuals with heart disease. As our understanding of biological systems grows, so will our ability to develop innovative therapies and strategies to address various health challenges. Medicine is increasingly relying on biological insights to optimise patient care and outcomes.

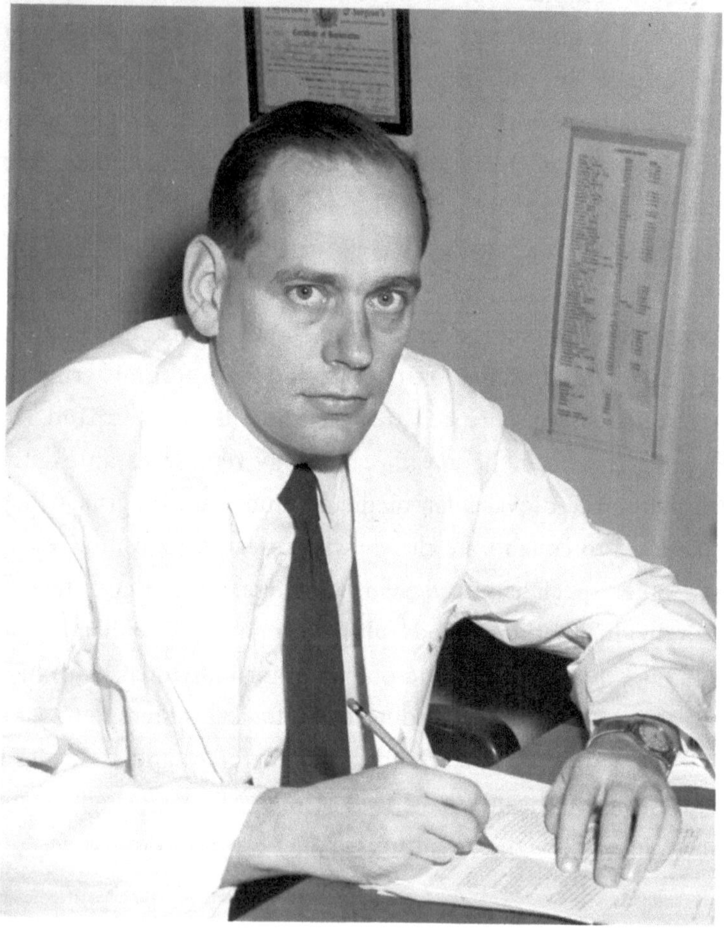

Chapter 5
Eugene Stead

Dr Eugene A. Stead Jr. (1908–2005) was an American physician and educator known for his significant contributions to medical education and internal medicine. He served at the Duke University School of Medicine as a professor for many years. Dr Eugene Stead's legacy is multifaceted and far-reaching, impacting medical education and healthcare delivery. I found Dr Stead's writings to be a beacon of medical education, which is the backbone of any country's healthcare delivery system and deeply embedded in society. Dr Stead was the first doctor of eminence to raise an alarm that medical schools operating in specialised areas, the apprenticeship, are no longer concerned with the patient's general care.

You can only enter a medical college if you pass a rigorously competitive qualifying examination. The journey to graduating from medical school lasts four and a half years and is followed by a mandatory one-year internship. Then comes post-graduation - becoming a specialist and super-specialist. Again, a medical graduate must compete to secure limited seats. That piece of parchment is relevant, indeed. Therefore, our country has a monopoly on creating skilled medical manpower in the hands of medical colleges. The question, then, is how much these colleges are primarily concerned with the patient's care. Even more fundamental than that is the question: Can anything be done to improve the system? This chapter searches for answers from his book *A Way of Working*[24] here.

First and foremost is the uniqueness of the medical profession, wherein it chooses the people who would enter the system. Today, students are admitted to medical college by a nationwide examination. And though there are some inclusive policies in place that favour candidates coming from disadvantageous groups in society, it is a merit-based process and there are no significant discrepancies in who can be a medical student except for being good in one's studies. But the reality of medical practice brings these worthy young people in touch with the sick and even poor patients. So, the most crucial part of their education is how to train them to deal with people – both patients and their anxious, and at times angry, attendants. Dr Stead says they are best taught by encouraging them to prepare themselves.

> Most medical educators would agree that the internship and residency are part of the doctor's educational program and that these years are best spent in a teaching hospital . . . I have always said that a teaching hospital is one in which the intern and resident can teach, rather than one in which they are taught. Medical students are the greatest single asset of a teaching hospital. Properly woven into the program,

24 Stead, E.A., Haynes, B.R. (editor), *A Way of Working: Essays on the Practice of Medicine*, Durham: Carolina Academic Press, 2001.

> they give the intern and resident the opportunity for an active participation in the learning, which can come only from establishing correlations between biologic processes and diseases from the manipulation of ideas and from the painting of word pictures. I know of many ways to teach medical students without the use of interns and residents as teachers. I know of no method of intern and resident training that is as effective as one that involves them directly in the teaching program. (p. 23)

Dr Stead is brilliant in describing the evolution of medical practice and education. He explains it as a symbiotic process and not separated. It is fashionable to see hospitals, especially the bigger ones, shape themselves as research institutes. Dr Stead declares 'education' as a medical college's primary function–converting untrained students into trained human resources. The patient services provided in a teaching hospital should be part of training the students. It must be clear to the authorities who control these organisations and the people teaching there, as well as the patients who choose to receive their treatments there.

> The primary output of a medical center is doctors; the primary output of a research institute is knowledge. The training of doctors to do research results in a higher unit cost for the new knowledge than one needs to pay if they are not teaching students. The medical centre may give excellent medical services in terms of the final product. It will not give these excellent services efficiently and at a low unit cost if they are an integral part of the education program . . . . The medical faculty is able to teach in the classroom, to teach in the research laboratory,

> and to teach in its hospitals and clinics because monies have been found to pay the faculty for its total educational effort. There is no magic in the system. Remove the money – stop paying for faculty time, require service to be given efficiently, and require the output of new knowledge to be the major goal of the laboratories to balance the budget: the medical centre will fail as an educational unit. (p. 32)

Dr Stead wrote the above passage in 1970. He was spot on in his observation. I have seen some great medical colleges failing due to lack of funds. The faculty were not paid adequately, so they resorted to part-time private practice rather than spending time teaching at the patient's bedside with their students. And society accepted it by rewarding them by patronising their private clinics rather than punishing them for this aberration. The opposite happened in the corporate hospitals, where everything was measured in terms of money, and hardly any research occurred there except sponsored clinical trials.

Dr Stead also cautioned against sending residents and interns to community hospitals. This would have robbed the young doctors of their golden period when they could have captured the theoretical underpinnings of medical practice in the company of their teachers. In the community hospitals, they would have become slaves to seeing the never-ending flow of patients and serving them routines dictated by the administration. What greater harm can any country do itself?

> The internship and residency are golden years in which one can learn both the medicine of today and the language and

> theoretical underpinning of the medicine of tomorrow. No community hospital has the faculty to combine these two elements—the best practice of today and the best preparation for the practice of tomorrow . . .
>
> The problem of the doctor practising in the community hospital cannot possibly be solved by the intern-resident model. The number of house staff required to staff this model is greatly in excess of the available total number of interns and residents . . . doctors in practice need a clinical support system, but the intern-resident support system does not meet their need. (p. 34)

In the mid-1960s, the United States faced a shortage of primary care physicians. Dr Stead conceived the idea of training non-physician healthcare workers to perform routine medical tasks under the supervision of physicians. This led to the development of the first Physician Assistants (PA) program at Duke University in 1965, which marked the beginning of the PA profession. Stead's vision and leadership played a crucial role in establishing the PA role as a valuable part of the healthcare system, providing accessible and high-quality patient care.

The primary goals of the PA profession are to expand access to healthcare services, particularly in underserved areas, and to improve the efficiency of healthcare delivery. PAs are trained to perform various medical tasks, including conducting physical exams, diagnosing and treating illnesses, ordering and interpreting diagnostic tests, prescribing medications, and providing patient education and counselling.

> The discovery by the doctor that his assistant can do any one day the majority of things that he himself does raises some interesting questions about medical education. Why does it take so long to educate the doctor and so little time to educate the assistant?
>
> The doctor's education system consists of four parts: (1) preparation to function as a citizen, (2) language preparation so that he can obtain content as needed from books written in part in symbolic languages, (3) development of problem-solving abilities, and (4) application of known knowledge to medical practice . . .
>
> The overall purpose of the long educational program for doctors is to prepare them for a lifetime of good citizenship and a lifetime of learning. The intent is to create thinking doctors who are completely protected against obsolescence regardless of changes in the societal and technological scene. (p. 35, 36)

The concept of Physician Assistants has evolved over the years, with the profession gaining recognition and acceptance as an integral part of the healthcare system. PAs play a crucial role in addressing the growing demand for healthcare services, particularly in primary care and other underserved areas, and contribute to improving access to quality healthcare for patients across the United States and in several different countries where the profession has been adopted.

During the Presidency of Dr APJ Abdul Kalam, I attempted to set up a Physician Assistant program suited for Indian conditions, where a large number of nurses and other technical people who seemed to be in a career rut were retrained as Physician Assistants. We joined with Netaji Subhas Open University to provide a graduate diploma to the PAs we trained based on the curriculum we jointly developed. The Emergency Management and Research Institute (EMRI) system brought in a PA program in collaboration with Stanford University, USA, and affiliated it with Osmania University, Hyderabad. The two-year Advanced PG Diploma in Emergency Care (APGDEC) was designed to develop world-class Emergency Medical Care Professionals. Later, I created the Care Institute of Health Sciences (CIHS) to institutionalise skill generation.

Skill generation in the hospital industry refers to developing and enhancing healthcare professionals' competencies, knowledge, and abilities to meet the evolving needs and challenges of the healthcare sector. Skill generation is essential for ensuring high-quality patient care, promoting innovation, and maintaining a competent workforce. Several key factors contribute to skill generation in the hospital industry, and I enlist seven here. These are needed and can be ignored only at the cost of operational efficiency.

1. **Education and Training Programs**: Hospitals invest in education and training programs to equip healthcare professionals with the knowledge and skills necessary to perform their roles effectively. This includes continuing education opportunities, workshops, seminars, and in-service training sessions to keep staff updated on the latest advancements in medical technology, treatments, and best practices.

2. **Clinical Experience and Hands-On Training:** Healthcare professionals, including doctors, nurses, technicians, and other staff, gain essential skills through hands-on clinical experience. Hospitals provide opportunities for professionals to work directly with patients under the supervision of experienced mentors, allowing them to apply theoretical knowledge in real-world healthcare settings.

3. **Specialized Training Programs:** Many hospitals offer training programs in various medical specialities and subspecialties to meet specific healthcare needs. These programs may include physician residency and fellowship programs, advanced practice nursing programs, and training programs for allied health professionals.

4. **Simulation and Technology-Based Training:** Simulation-based training using high-fidelity mannequins, virtual reality simulations, and other technology-enhanced learning tools allows healthcare professionals to practice clinical skills and scenarios in a controlled environment. These training methods help improve clinical decision-making, teamwork, and communication skills while minimising patient risks.

5. **Interdisciplinary Collaboration:** Hospitals foster interdisciplinary collaboration among healthcare professionals from different disciplines, such as physicians, nurses, pharmacists, therapists, and social workers. Collaborative practice environments encourage

knowledge sharing, skill development, and the exchange of best practices across disciplines, ultimately enhancing patient care outcomes.

6. **Quality Improvement Initiatives:** Hospitals implement quality improvement initiatives to identify areas for skill improvement and implement strategies to enhance clinical performance and patient safety. Continuous quality improvement efforts involve ongoing monitoring, evaluation, and feedback mechanisms to drive skill generation and professional development.

7. **Leadership Development:** Hospitals invest in leadership development programs to cultivate leadership skills among healthcare professionals at all organisational levels. Leadership training helps individuals effectively manage teams, drive organisational change, and foster a culture of innovation and excellence.

Overall, skill generation in the hospital industry is a dynamic and multifaceted process that requires a commitment to lifelong learning, continuous improvement, and collaboration among healthcare professionals, educators, and healthcare organisations. By investing in skill generation initiatives, hospitals can strengthen their workforce, improve patient outcomes, and adapt to the evolving healthcare landscape.

The second thing I learnt from Dr Stead was about the purpose of life. His essay *Paid in Full by the Satisfaction of Each Day*, published in 1973, touched my heart. I lived my professional life according to the unvarying characteristics of Dr Stead's vision of medicine and the world. I quote three passages from the essay from his biography *The Doctors' Doctor.*[25] The first passage relates to children, and I don't know how much my two sons suffered by me following this.

> The Past is gone; the future may never be attained. The present is real, tangible, and waits to be enjoyed. In my professional life, I have never spent a year with any other purpose than to enjoy the year. If the year advanced my career, that was an additional bonus; if it did not, I lost nothing because I had been paid in full by the satisfaction of each day . . . The realization that the returns from living are collected each day does modify one's behaviour. One is unwilling to sacrifice everything in the present for something in future . . .
>
> As the children grew older, we made it clear that we would support them until they were able to support themselves. After that, we would expect to see them and their children. If all of us enjoyed the venture. When they were capable of independence, we owed them nothing and they owed us nothing. We have collected our pleasures as we want, and there were no debts.

The second passage is about professional life. In India, doctors have traditionally been regarded highly by society. The present impression of private business-mindedness of some in the profession has led to a poor image of doctors. One factor

25 Laszlo, John, Neelon Francis A., *The Doctor's Doctor: A Biography of Eugene A. Stead Jr., MD*, Carolina Academic Press, 2006.

contributing to this poor image of doctors is the sensationalization of every news item, often ignoring information that glosses over mundane details, exonerating a doctor in an incident of alleged medical negligence.

There are two aspects. As a hypothetical example, a television reporter shouting at the medical superintendent of a Delhi hospital reeling under a load of dengue patients as to why antimalarials were not given to a patient who died of dengue. This is done with an air of 'knowledge' that viewers would be convinced that not giving antimalarials to a patient with dengue was medical negligence of the highest order. But equally serious is the issue of overreach. Modern medicine is changing rapidly. Hence, attempting to treat and perform procedures beyond the scope of one's training and facilities is inappropriate. Remaining within one's capability and experience is more critical than ever. All clinical establishments must develop an SOP for handling violence against medical staff by patient attendants, and politicians must stay away from protecting hooligans in the larger interest of the medical profession and the public that it eventually serves.

> A doctor cannot treat disease. He must care for the patient who has the disease. The doctor who wakes each morning with zest for the adventures of the day is at peace with his patients. He knows the limits that the structure of the nervous system puts on the behaviour of the people. He doesn't expect all things from all men. He can comfortably make fewer demands on persons who, because of genetic background, unfavourable environment, ignorance, fear, or prejudice, have ceilings on their performance. The doctor who enjoys

> the day develops a high degree of tolerance for the frailties of man and enjoys to the fullest the triumph of individuals. The educational program chosen by the young doctor should be one that teaches him to enjoy the people who have the illnesses he is learning to treat. That is the only way to assure that the work of each day will bring true satisfaction.

The third passage is about the social life. The role of the doctor continues to evolve as society changes. From being an authoritarian figure practising in an autocratic and often isolated way, the doctor's role has changed to one where partnership with patients is the cornerstone of the relationship. Advances in science and technology, including increased use of the Internet and the increasingly multidisciplinary approach to healthcare, have also contributed to the changing relationship. The medical profession has to understand that professionalism and its obligations are the basis of society's expectations.

> Many times the social structure is so tight that only penalties accrue as change occurs. A young man starting his career may be able to offer many contributions . . . He may begin as an excellent bio scientist. Later as clinical interest becomes stronger, he becomes an increasingly important clinician . . . in due course he becomes an outstanding leader in his area of clinical specialization and devotes more time to national affairs. This evolution requires a flexible system of funding so that the person can be supported from different sources as his functions change.

A layperson would like to believe that most doctors are greedy professionals who wish to live and work in urban areas for monetary benefits or worldly pleasures. But then the evidence is otherwise. There is no campus interview for any level of medical qualification at any medical institution in India, including the All India Institute of Medical Sciences (AIIMS). The average salary of a fresh medical graduate (MBBS) at private hospitals in metros like Bengaluru, Hyderabad, Chennai and Mumbai is much lower than an entry-level IT industry employee. In most cities, this income cannot support even a lower-middle-class standard of living. For every superstar medical professional, there are a hundred strugglers and a thousand toiling in despair, no better than indentured labourers of the colonial past in their free country.

The majority of doctors do not have any forum to voice their concerns. Their issues often need to be more represented by proxy leaders. The professional fraternity is getting more and more structured like hierarchical pyramids with few super specialists, which are, in fact, sub-specialities at the top and a large number of primary care physicians at the bottom. General practitioners, family physicians, medical officers, resident medical officers, and recently qualified medical graduates - are disfranchised from academic and professional leadership positions. Medical professionals are compartmentalised into rigid occupational vocations. The vocational training and long-term career paths for primary care doctors have been blocked at the regulatory level.

By 2030, India will have one million additional MBBS doctors; currently, 50,000 are added annually. Contrary to the perception of scarcity of medical doctors, a large section of newly qualified physicians are spending considerable years in dysfunctional status due to mismanagement of human resources in the healthcare system as it functions in India. There are very few employment opportunities for qualified doctors in the public sector; simultaneously, the average salary of MBBS doctors in urban private hospitals is meagre. Paradoxically, there is no actual demand for medical professionals in a country of more than 1.4 billion people. While the popular perception is that young doctors are not willing to do community service, a reality check is required on the public sector's and industry's intent and capacity towards engaging medical doctors in the service delivery process.

Due to aggressive unregulated business practices of the medical industry, mostly corporatised and owned by faceless investors committed to return on investment, an environment for malpractice and corruption has been created for the industrial consumption of pharmaceutical and consumable medical products. Physicians and doctors who used to be trusted partners of the patients and communities are losing faith in the people. Their position to negotiate on behalf of the ordinary people has been severely compromised. Instead of taking professional calls, the existing proxy leaders of the medical profession are busy defending their positions and can maintain the status quo. For how long this will continue? There is a barefaced leadership vacuum in the Indian medical profession, and young doctors are toiling in despair if someone cares to find out.

Finally, I must mention Dr Stead's fitness and zeal to work even in his nineties. Time marches on, Dr Stead has famously said. And that there are three causes of illness - made wrong, worn out, and bad luck—one life to become old by making it past that juggernaut. As average life expectancy steadily rises, people live longer and more actively. In the 21st century, becoming elderly is to be expected, and it's a good, everyday thing. But what about the "frail elderly"? That is obviously not a good thing.

The definition of "frail elderly" includes at least three clinical features: loss of strength, weight loss, low levels of activity, poor endurance or fatigue, and slowed performance. Frailty may be secondary, in which case the patient also has a recognised and diagnosed severe disease, such as cancer, stroke, COPD, heart failure, liver failure, psychosis, or dementia. But even without any disease present the patient can be "frail" nonetheless.

There is an increasing need and demand for long-term care in the people's home environment. Such care aims to allow people to stay at home and avoid hospitalisation or other institutional care. In-home health care must be provided at the highest possible quality, focusing on people's needs and experiences. The CIHS had developed an elderly-focused PA program with quality of care as the central theme. There are three categories and seven subcategories related to frail older people's needs and experiences of home health care.

The first category, Safe and Secure Care, consisted of three subcategories: Education and Experience of Nurses, Information, and Continuity of Care regarding personnel continuity and regular care. The second category, Autonomy, contained two subcategories: Decision-making and Self-sufficiency. The last category, Relationship with Professionals, consisted of two subcategories: Personality of Nurse and Partnerships. We need to revamp the healthcare industry with skilled people. A new generation of Physician Assistants must be groomed to hone the skills of assisting doctors the way they need it – from nursing to office to research assistant to undertaking outreach work autonomously as an extension of the physician on the other end.

Dr Stead's vision for Physician Assistants was to create healthcare providers to help bridge the gap between doctors and patients, ultimately improving access to quality healthcare. Structuring Pas' education and utilising them can be a cost-effective way for hospitals to manage patient loads, as PAs can often provide high-quality care at a lower cost than physicians. The ideal education mix for Physician Assistants should typically include a Bachelor's Degree and an accredited PA program. The perfect education mix for Physician Assistants consists of a strong foundation in science and a commitment to be in the healthcare sector for a lifetime.

Ideally, after completing a PA program, graduates must pass a Physician Assistant National Certifying Exam. However, this exam is not even available for doctors and nurses in India, so it is left to their councils and employers. PA must complete several clinical hours in various healthcare settings, such as hospitals, clinics, and primary care offices. This hands-on experience is essential for developing practical skills and exposure to medical specialities. Once employed, they must participate in continuing education activities to maintain their certification and stay current with advances in healthcare. This ongoing professional development is crucial for ensuring the delivery of high-quality patient care.

Physician's Assistants' versatility, adaptability, and comprehensive medical training make them valuable healthcare providers in various settings and specialisations. PAs have diverse opportunities outside of traditional hospital services. In primary care settings, PAs can provide preventive care, diagnose and treat common illnesses, and manage chronic conditions under the supervision of a physician. PAs are well-suited to work in urgent care settings, where they can see patients with acute but non-life-threatening conditions, order tests, prescribe medications, and provide necessary treatments. PAs play a vital role in community health centres, serving underserved populations, promoting health education, and addressing the healthcare needs of diverse communities.

Anganwadi workers are frontline community health workers crucial in delivering primary healthcare and nutrition services to women and children in rural and urban communities. They are typically responsible for essential services such as immunisation, preschool education, maternal and child healthcare, and nutrition support. While both Anganwadi workers and Physician Assistants contribute to healthcare delivery, their roles, responsibilities, and training requirements are distinct. Anganwadi workers focus on community-based health promotion and primary healthcare services. Physician Assistants engage in clinical practice and deliver a broader scope of medical care under the guidance of licensed physicians.

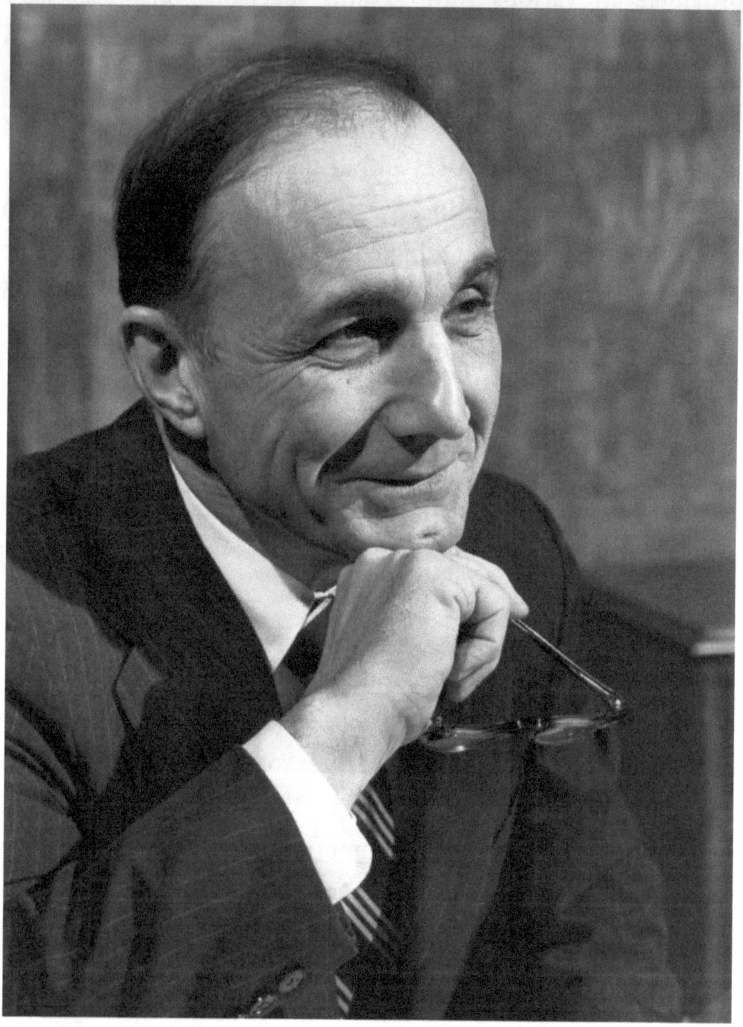

Chapter 6
Edmund Pellegrino

Dr Pellegrino is the final figure among those great doctors who inspired me and shaped my thoughts. American physician, ethicist, and academic Edmund Daniel Pellegrino (1920 –2013) was a prominent figure in bioethics. Throughout his career, he advocated for a humanistic approach to medicine, emphasising the importance of compassion, integrity, and the primacy of the patient's welfare. Dr Pellegrino served as the Chairman of the President's Council on Bioethics under President George W. Bush from 2005 to 2009.

Cardiology embraced modern technology in the late 1990s with the digitisation of echocardiography and Cath labs. Until the 1960s, the available Myocardial Infarction (MI) treatments mainly were palliative rather than interventional. Although the introduction of coronary care units in the 1970s brought down the early mortality rate significantly, a more effective method to treat MI, directed at its very cause, was required. A "wonder drug" was needed to dissolve the clot, triggering MI.

Just like the musk deer wander their entire lives searching for the arcane source of musk, not knowing that the fragrance emanates from their bodies, what cardiologists were looking for had already been discovered years ago. In the 1930s, a professor of medicine at the New York University School of Medicine, William Tillett (1892-1974), had observed that streptococci agglutinated in test tubes that contained human plasma, but not in those that contained human serum. Tillett inferred that the agglutination of streptococci was caused by a component of plasma deficient in serum.

The prime candidate for this agglutinating activity was fibrinogen. Tillett further hypothesised that fibrinogen is adsorbed onto the surface of streptococci, rendering the plasma devoid of free fibrinogen. This led to the knowledge that any plasma containing streptococci would not clot because it would lack free fibrinogen, a key clotting factor. But tinkering with fibrinogen is fraught with pyrogenic reactions that could be fatal.

In contrast to the situation in the 1960s and 1970s, the mortality risk for patients with myocardial infarction has been reduced, particularly for those with myocardial infarction with cardiogenic shock (MICS). Approximately 5-10 % of patients with a myocardial infarction are affected by a MICS, and the mortality risk is between 30 % and 50 %. The primary percutaneous coronary intervention with stent implantation should be carried out as quickly as possible to reduce the mortality to around 20%. It was nothing short of a revolution.

The scion of Siris Pharmaceutical, Rama Raju, established a biotech company, Sudarshan Biotech. He was guided by renowned scientist Prof Ramareddy Guntaka, who was working at the University of Tennessee Health Science Center College of Medicine, established perhaps the first biotechnology platform in India. But later, the biotechnology industry was overtaken by the Hepatitis vaccine excitement and the money it brought. A clot-specific streptokinase (CSSK) finally arrived at the Institute of Microbial Technology (IMTECH), Chandigarh, only in the 2010s by Dr Girish Sahni and his team.

By this time, biotechnology has been revolutionising medicine in numerous ways. It was realised that biotechnology allows for the customisation of medical treatments based on an individual's genetic makeup, lifestyle, and environment. This approach can lead to more effective treatments with fewer side effects. It is possible to develop targeted therapies that attack disease-causing molecules or cells, minimising damage to healthy tissue, reducing side effects and improving patient outcomes. Techniques like CRISPR-Cas9 enable precise editing of genes, offering potential cures for genetic diseases.

A new era in Medicine had begun and it needed a modern Hippocrates. Dr Pellegrino assumed that role and won worldwide acceptance. He contributed significantly to the philosophy of medicine, exploring the nature of illness, healing, and the physician-patient relationship. His writings delved into the fundamental values and principles that underpin medical practice and I share here some passages from Dr Pellrgrino's *The Philosophy of Medicine Reborn*,[26] reminding us of the enduring

26 Pellegrino, E.D., Engelhardt, H.T., (editor), Fabrice Jotterand (editor), *The Philosophy of Medicine Reborn: A Pellgrino Reader*, Notre Dame: University of Notre Dame Press, 2011.

importance of ethical reflection and moral integrity in healthcare. I have selected three themes – who controls medicine, the doctor-patient relationship, and expanding medical ethics.

The first and foremost question medicine faces today is whether it should be teleologically or socially constructed. The dilemma is whether medicine is something as a function of its end or as a function of its cause, that is, illness and diseases. And does society have the power to decide what it should be? As biotechnology and artificial intelligence change the fundamentals of human life and health, it becomes the central question of our time.

> A teleologically oriented philosophy of medicine is certainly not a Doctor- or patient-defined entity. The very notion of a reality-based philosophy of medicine contravenes any idea that physicians or patients determine what medicine is. Rather, physicians do what they do and patients act as they do because both are pursuing an end in which they are joined by the realities of being ill, being healed, and professing to heal. The moral pursuit of these relationships is what determines what is right and good. The "good" . . . is a compound notion in which medicine, the patients, and the good of humans and for humans are closely interrelated. (p. 53)
>
> There is already a move among some ethicists, economists, and policymakers to redirect physicians from a person-centered to a society-centered ethic. The purpose is to preserve resources by relieving the physician of her traditional primary commitment to act for the welfare of her

> patient. Medical ethics in this way would become socially constructed in accord with the canon of economics rather than the personal obligation of doctors to their patients. The primacy of the sick person is thus to be displaced by the needs of distant, unidentified, possible future patients according to some schema of social worth. (p. 58)

Good clinical expertise gathers the best available evidence and—most importantly—considers patients' preferences and values. The medication must be moderated to minimise side effects, and diet and lifestyle approaches must be widely deployed. Has our healthcare system failed to adhere to this gold standard of clinical practice for the most critical goal of improving patient health outcomes? Some thinkers believe that modern medicine, through over-prescription, represents a significant threat to public health.

In my view, the cost of an ageing population is not a threat to the welfare system - an unhealthy ageing population is. Managing almost entirely preventable chronic conditions such as heart disease, high blood pressure, and type 2 diabetes holds the key. Type 2 diabetes can be reversed in up to half of the patients by refraining from sugar consumption and doing exercise. Yet rather than addressing the root cause of these conditions through lifestyle changes, we prioritise drugs that give, at best, only a marginal chance of long-term benefit for individuals, most of whom will derive no health outcome improvement.

But who will take responsibility for spreading awareness? The media is run by businesses selling carbonated sugary syrups and mostly useless supplements. Even alcohol and tobacco are peddled through clever surrogate advertisements, and top film stars promote them without any shame.

The reality is that lifestyle changes reduce the risk of future disease, but their positive effects on quality of life can be experienced within days to weeks. However, those patients unlucky enough to suffer side effects from prescribed medicines may find their quality of life will deteriorate to enjoy small, longer-term benefits from the medication. It can be done only by practising doctors to promote their patient's healthy lifestyles rather than putting them on prescription drugs as a habit. How are ordinary people expected to know what is good for them? It's never too late to improve fitness. You can never be healthy by keeping on medicines.

Dr Amartya Sen wrote an insightful article around the turn of the millennium that addresses the dilemma head-on.

> Critical scrutiny of public health care and medical strategy depends, among other things, on how individual states of health and illness are assessed . . . there is a conceptual contrast between "internal" views of health (based on the patient's perceptions) and "external" views (based on the observations of doctors or pathologists). Although the two views can certainly be combined (a good practitioner would be interested in both), major tension often exists between evaluations based respectively on the two perspectives . . . . There is a strong need for scrutinising the statistics on self-perception of illness in a social context by taking note of levels of education, availability of health facilities, and public

> information on illness and remedy . . . The internal view of health deserves attention, but relying on it in assessing health care or in evaluating medical strategy can be extremely misleading.[27]

Dr Pellegrino emphasized the need for a better Doctor-Patient relationship in the light of four principles of maleficence, beneficence, autonomy, and justice – celebrated as tetrad par excellence – and used doctors and ethicists to resolve ethical dilemmas and define the right conduct of doctors and patients. Dr Pellegrino argued that the four principles should never be abandoned.

> Briefly, the ends of medicine are ultimately the restoration or improvement of health, and more proximately, to heal, i.e., to cure illness or disease or, when this is not possible, to care for and help the patient to live with residual pain, discomfort, or disability. There are many decisions along the way to these ends, but in each decision, there is a fusion of technical and moral agreements. If it were merely a matter of technical correctness, of medical good alone, the major moral principle would be competence . . . but the doctor will use her promised competence not for her own ends but for those of the patient and . . . efface her own interests in respect of the patient. i.e., the promises to serve the patient's good. But this good is more than simple medical good; it includes the patient's perception of good, material, emotional, or spiritual. (p. 200)

27 https://www.ncbi.nlm.nih.gov/pmc/articles/PMC1122815/. Last accessed on March 15, 2024.

> On the view I am taking, the four principles are derived from obligations owned by doctors. These obligations, in turn, derive from the promise to provide competent help, which is at the heart of the medical relationship. The primary obligation that unifies the theory of medical ethics is beneficence—beneficence not mistakenly equated with paternalism, but beneficence-in-trust, beneficence which fuses respect for the person of the patient with the obligation not just to prevent or remove harm, but to do good. The primary obligation is not non-maleficence, which is a negative obligation required even by law. Beneficence requires preventing harm, removing harm, and doing good even at some cost and risk to oneself. Thus there is an implicit promise of some degree of self-effacement of the doctor's interests in favour of the patient's interests. (p. 201)

Expanding medical ethics is the need of the hour. According to Dr Pellegrino, the Hippocratic principle of primum non nocere must be expanded to encompass the patient's value system to be genuine in the modern world. Ironically, with so many advances in science and technology, the concept of "health" as a positive entity is as vague today as in Hippocrates' time. Its definition is highly personal, and the physician's view of health may be quite at variance with that of the patient or society.

> Indeed, society must set its own priorities for health. The amelioration of social disorders like alcoholism, sociopathy, drug addiction, and violence can have greater value for a healthy human existence, for example, than merely

> prolonging life in patients with chronic disabling disorders . . . The configuration of value choices each of us makes defines concretely our uniqueness and individuality . . . Physicians are also individuals with sets of values which invariably colour their professional acts. Their views of sex, alcohol, suffering, poverty, race, and so forth can sharply differ with those of their patients . . . Physicians must constantly guard against confusing their own values as the "good" to which all must subscribe if they desire to be treated by them. (p. 407)

> Even more vexing questions in social ethics are posed when we attempt to allocate our resources among the many new possibilities for good inherent in medical progress and technology. Do we pool our limited resources and manpower to apply curative medicine to all now deprived of it or continue to multiply the complexity of services for the privileged? Do we apply mass prophylaxis against streptococcal disease, or repair damaged valves with expensive heart surgery? Is it preferable to change cultural patterns in favour of a more reasonable diet . . . or develop better surgical techniques for unplugging fat-occluded coronary arteries? Every health planner and concerned public official has his or her own set of similar questions. It is clear that we cannot have all these things simultaneously. (p, 408)

One common theme of my life has been my continued interaction with medical students. They somehow reached out to me, and I always encouraged them and took classes that were more focused on ethics and what is good for doctors and the profession. I have no hesitation in declaring that our young doctors are now increasingly suffering from "demoralisation syndrome," characterised by a sense of helplessness and loss of purpose. The demoralisation is not a reaction to their workload but is caused by the diseased systems we work for. During the Covid-19 pandemic, the consequences of a lousy system have intensified, and many young doctors have been left shaken. Hearing from a young PG that being a doctor in a broken place required a belief that the place would become less broken due to their efforts was an eye-opener as it was painful. Had my generation of doctors collectively failed?

It has become fashionable to talk about being overworked: burnout. Nearly half the physicians report they are experiencing its symptoms. I'm afraid I have to disagree. I know from my personal experience what it means to do multiple shifts, prepare for exams, and manage inadequacy or shortage of almost everything, even electricity outages at times. To me, the burnout rhetoric misses the more significant issue in this case: What's burning out healthcare workers is less the gruelling conditions they practice under and more our dwindling faith in the systems for which they work. What has been identified as occupational burnout is a symptom of a more profound collapse. We are witnessing the slow death of medical ideology, which is unfortunate.

When I sit with my old professional friends over a drink in the evening, and we bring our experiences out on the table, not as memories but feelings, it reveals how our belief system is made up of interlinking political, moral, and cultural narratives upon which we depend to make sense of our social world. Faith in the traditional stories we have told about ourselves, stories that have long sustained what should have been an unsustainable system, is now dissolving. During the pandemic, young doctors witnessed our hospitals nearly fall apart due to underinvestment in public health systems and uneven distribution of medical infrastructure. Long-ignored inequalities in the standard of care available to the rich and poor became front-page news as bodies were stacked in empty hospital rooms and makeshift morgues. Many healthcare workers have been traumatised by the futility of their attempts to stem recurrent waves of death, with nearly one-fifth of physicians reporting they knew a colleague who had considered, attempted, or died by suicide during the first year of the pandemic alone.

Resistance to self-criticism has long been a hallmark of the medical profession and the industry it has shaped. Political leaders lauded "socialised medicine" but have repeatedly defended health care as a business venture by incentivising patients to receive treatment in private hospitals instead of strengthening public institutions. It has become such a menace that no one gained in the end except perhaps the corrupt officials, who always lived insignificant lives of parasites in every era. Private hospitals have brought good medical care to India when government hospitals failed. Enormous investments and business risks were taken to make India good at attracting international patients. For a profession that had fought for more than a century to achieve elite status, this was a great thing to happen, and many great doctors shifted to the private sector, looking for the professional autonomy and resourcefulness that eluded them in the government hospital, and make less money.

However, the young doctors who beelined to work in the private sector as soon they completed their PG accreditation soon learned to rationalise a deeply unequal health care system that emphasises personal, rather than public, moral responsibility for protecting health. They sit at their patients' bedsides and counsel them on their duty to counteract the risks of obesity, heart disease and diabetes, for example, while largely ignoring how those diseases are tied to their inappropriate lifestyles. Part of what draws us into this norm is that doctors learn by doing — that is, via apprenticeship — in which we repeat what's modelled for us. This is, to a degree, a necessary aspect of training in an applied technical field. It is also a fundamentally conservative model for learning that teaches us to suppress critical thinking and trust the system, even with its perverse incentives. It becomes difficult to recognise the origins of much of what we do and whose interests it serves. For example, a system of billing codes invented by insurance companies as part of a business strategy now dictates nearly every aspect of medical practice, producing endless administrative work and subtly shaping treatment choices.

Addressing the healthcare system's failures will require uncomfortable reflection and bold action. Any illusion that medicine and politics are, or should be, separate spheres has been crushed under the weight of people killed in a pandemic that was, in many ways, should have been a manageable, if not preventable, disaster. And many physicians are now finding it difficult to quash the suspicion that our institutions, and much of our work inside them, primarily serve a moneymaking machine. Can doctors be passive witnesses to these harms? Don't we have a responsibility to use our collective power to insist on changes: universal health care, paid sick leave, investments in community health worker programs, and essential housing and social welfare systems?

Will the Indian Medical Association (IMA), a century-old system, be able to build the systems it needs to be true to its profession? Someday, we must face the unpleasant truth that our healthcare institutions as they exist today are part of the problem rather than the solution. Here, Pellegrino's legacy embodies a commitment to compassion, humanism, and the importance of the patient's welfare in medical practice. He emphasised the importance of treating each patient as unique and deserving of respect and dignity.

Competency is the prime quality of a doctor. With the scientific era in medicine, the efficacy of new techniques and information in changing the natural history of disease is dramatically demonstrated. Today, patients can access new knowledge. The increasing number of them come armed with medicines' names and procedure details. Side effects are discussed more than the treatment. Maintaining competence today is the prime ethical challenge a doctor faces. There is no question that all 21st-century healthcare professionals must thoroughly understand the benefits and limitations of AI, and they are likely to use it extensively in their clinical work. These include skills in using the electronic health record (EHR), accessing clinical knowledge using search systems, being facile with clinical decision support and health information exchange, protecting privacy and security, engaging patients, their data, and their devices, and applying data in tasks such as population health, public health, and clinical and translational research. These competencies provide a foundation for using data, information, and knowledge to improve human health and healthcare delivery. Still, they also inform the application of AI in biomedicine and health.

However, another area of required competence has come to the fore in recent years: the paroxysmal arrival of machine learning and artificial/augmented intelligence in medicine. While these impacts in real-world clinical practice are still minor, the long-term effect will likely be substantial. Indeed, clinicians should be familiar with the myriad of issues related to algorithms and models, including ethical concerns. As we see biotechnology and artificial intelligence creating possibilities that were not even imaginable, and real-time monitoring using mobile phones as a platform and AI-powered alerts giving patients new tools of self-preservation, Dr Pellegrino's writings continue to inspire ongoing discussions and debates in the fields of medicine and bioethics, reminding us of the enduring importance of ethical reflection and moral integrity in healthcare.

As more people embrace modern medicine, the shift from traditional to modern medicine raises important bioethical considerations impacting patient care, healthcare delivery, and societal values. Some key bioethical issues to consider in this transition include cultural sensitivity and integrative medicine. Modern medicine must respect and incorporate cultural beliefs, practices, and values from traditional medicine to ensure patient-centred care that is culturally sensitive and respectful of diverse backgrounds. The transition to modern medicine raises ethical questions about resource allocation, access to healthcare services, and equitable distribution of resources, particularly in underserved communities where traditional healing practices may still play a significant role.

There is growing interest in integrative medicine, which combines traditional and modern approaches to healthcare. Bioethics integrates healing modalities while upholding patient rights, safety, and well-being. In India, yoga therapy is often recommended to reduce stress, increase flexibility, and manage various health conditions such as anxiety, depression, and chronic pain. Good plant-based remedies such as herbs, roots, and flowers are available to support health and treat various ailments. Doctors may recommend herbal remedies alongside conventional treatments for insomnia, digestive disorders, and immune support. Integrative cardiologists may recommend supplements such as omega-3 fatty acids, Coenzyme Q10, and garlic for their anti-inflammatory, antioxidant, and cholesterol-lowering properties.

I close this chapter with an unresolved ethical issue here. A do-not-resuscitate (DNR) order is a legal document in the Western world, meaning a person has decided not to have cardiopulmonary resuscitation (CPR) attempted on them if their heart or breathing stops. People who choose to have a DNR usually have a terminal illness or other serious medical condition. The Do Not Resuscitate (DNR) order still needs to be documented in legal practice in India. It is a verbal communication between the clinician and the patient's relative or caregiver. There are guidelines, but the law needs to be more active and clear on most issues related to end-of-life care, and public awareness is created.

"I have made this thoughtful book by Dr. Lown required reading for physicians in the Program in Integrative Medicine at the University of Arizona. It conveys the wisdom about the doctor-patient relationship that has indeed been lost in the noise of high-tech, profit-driven medicine."
—ANDREW WEIL, M.D.

THE LOST ART OF HEALING

PRACTICING COMPASSION IN MEDICINE

"BERNARD LOWN...WRITES POWERFULLY OF THE MYSTERY AND MAJESTY OF MEDICINE."
—*The New York Times Book Review*

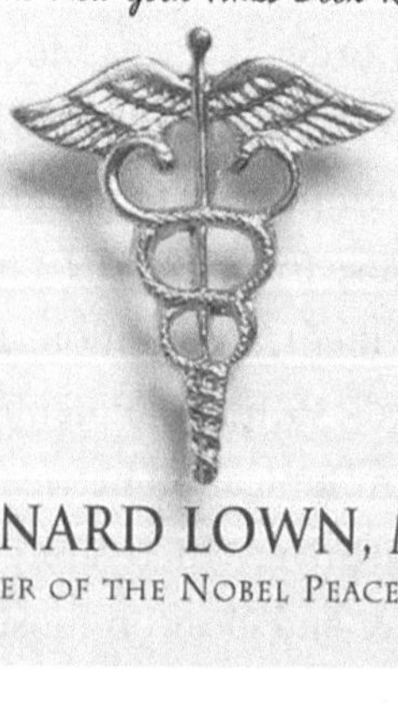

BERNARD LOWN, M.D.

WINNER OF THE NOBEL PEACE PRIZE

Chapter 7
The Lost Art of Healing

From this chapter onwards, the book takes up four themes: the personal interaction between doctor and patient, the transformation of the medical profession, how doctors remain passionate about their work, and the emergence of the healthcare system science of which doctors are a part. The pioneer of modern health care, Dr William Osler, emphasised the need for a humane bond that a doctor cultivates with patients. Dr Harrison further emphasised the human aspect of medicine, which became a creed.

This chapter is based on *The Lost Art of Healing: Practicing Compassion in Medicine*, a book by cardiologist Bernard Lown (1921 - 2021), published in 1996. It emphasises the importance of empathy and human connection in medical care. Dr Lown was best known for inventing the direct-current defibrillator and for his pioneering work in the field of cardiology. He co-founded the International Physicians for the Prevention of Nuclear War (IPPNW) in 1980, an organisation that won the Nobel Peace Prize in 1985.

The book emphasises that compassion is fundamental to healing and should be central to medical practice. Illness has inseparable emotional and psychological dimensions, and medical professionals must cultivate empathy and understanding for their patients. Dr Lown highlights the therapeutic value of listening to patients, acknowledging their fears and concerns, and involving them in decision-making processes.

Then, there is the holistic approach to medicine that considers the physical aspects of illness and the emotional, social, and spiritual dimensions. He believes addressing these broader health aspects is essential for promoting healing and well-being. While acknowledging the benefits of medical technology, Lown warns against the overreliance on technology at the expense of human interaction and compassion. He suggests that the impersonal nature of modern healthcare systems can lead to a loss of trust and satisfaction among patients.

The book also calls for reforms in healthcare systems to prioritise patient-centred care and restore the human touch to medicine. Policies that support continuity of care encourage interdisciplinary collaboration and foster a culture of compassion within medical institutions are paramount. Overall, *The Lost Art of Healing* is a poignant reminder of the importance of compassion, empathy, and human connection in medicine, urging healthcare professionals to rekindle these essential qualities in their work.

There is both mystery and majesty in medicine. It may sound poetic, but it explains medicine as a mystical scientific art. There is science as the backdrop of medicine - essential facts that reveal how physiology is disturbed during illness. Yet there are uncertainties - and quite many of them - about what triggers specific problems in the body and how it responds to the drugs and other interventions. When we say each individual is unique, it is not some cliché but a simple truth that every doctor knows. A good clinician is one who, by listening to the patient and doing a clinical examination, captures the uniqueness and fine-tunes his treatment.

Medicine has a vital spiritual component as it delves into the mysteries of life, health, and the human body. Despite remarkable advances in scientific understanding, countless aspects of health and disease still need to be completed. The human body's complexity, the intricacies of diseases, and the nuances of individual responses to treatment all contribute to the ongoing mystery of medicine. Additionally, there is the mystery of the human experience itself—our emotions and consciousness and their profound impact on health and healing.

The majesty of medicine encompasses the awe-inspiring achievements of medical science and practice. From developing life-saving vaccines to groundbreaking surgical procedures, medicine can transform lives and alleviate suffering. Moreover, the commitment and compassion of healthcare professionals who tirelessly dedicate themselves to the care of others embody the majesty of medicine. The profound sense of purpose and the noble pursuit of healing elevate medicine to a realm of majesty.

Together, the mystery and majesty of medicine encapsulate its enigmatic nature and its profound impact on humanity.

This interpretation underscores the awe-inspiring journey of discovery, compassion, and innovation that defines the practice of medicine. In my practice, I noticed that there is something inside every patient that was capable of reducing postoperative pain, boosting the survival chance of cancer patients, lowering the mortality rate in high-risk cardiac patients, and cutting the hospitalisation rate for diabetics.

Dr Lown best represents a scientific mind open to mysticism. He accepts the limitations of medicine, the indomitable life force, and its capacity to heal. He begins his book by invoking Hippocrates for the feeling of love for humanity at the core of the medical profession and German physician of the sixteenth century Paracelsus for intuition as the basic qualification of doctors to understand the patient, his body, and his disease. Intuition is indeed a sympathetic communication with the patient's spirit and does not involve any language or speech.

> I am convinced that listening beyond the chief complaint is the most effective, quickest, and least costly way to get to the bottom of most medical problems . . . 75 per cent of the information leading to a correct diagnosis comes from a detailed history, 10 per cent from the physical examination, 5 per cent from simple routine tests, 5 per cent from all the costly invasive tests, in 5 per cent, no answer is forthcoming. (p. 16)
>
> History-taking is always improved when another member of the family, especially a spouse, is present. Most doctors prefer to see patients alone, explaining that it is easier to focus on essentials and retain control. Another

> justification is that a patient alone is less inhibited. Intimate problems can be addressed which would otherwise remain undiscovered. (p. 18)
>
> I don't agree . . . such a presence speeds rather than impedes the flow of important information and shortens the time required to get to know the patient. Most important, a couple provides insight about family dynamics not really conveyed with words. By listening to the patient's responses and watching the spouse, one is immediately alerted to areas of potential trouble. Is the marriage successful or are they at each other throats? Is there a skeleton in a family closet? Are there conflicts with children? Is the patient's job too frustrating . . . These and many other problems are quickly brought to light when husband and wife are together. (p. 18-19)

Marital discord has been linked to both depression and anxiety; however, our understanding of how marriage contributes to the development of internalising symptoms is limited in scope and lacking specificity. First, it is unclear whether the marital relationship contributes to the broad dimension of internalising symptoms as opposed to specific diagnoses. Second, it is unclear how the marriage relationship contributes to internalising symptoms through global marital dissatisfaction or specific relationship processes. In my view, asymmetry in power and control is a risk factor for men regardless of the direction of the asymmetry. In contrast, low levels of emotional intimacy represent a risk factor for women. The irony is that remaining single in life has its plethora of problems.

From the dawn of medicine, physicians have been aware that emotions can predispose a person to disease as well as affect its outcome. Cardiologists have learned that psychological stresses can influence the most intimate aspects of heart function. Behavioural stresses may speed the heart rate, raise blood pressure, reduce coronary artery blood flow, enhance the electrical irritability of the heart, and change the contractile properties of the myocardium, the muscle that pumps the blood. In fact, a perturbed mind can disrupt heart rhythm, predispose to angina pectoris, precipitate a heart attack, and provoke sudden cardiac death. (p. 29)

Thus, history-taking involves not merely learning about a disease, but grasping what is agitating a patient's mind . . . Until the late nineteenth century, the mind was regarded as inseparable from the body, but as science gained dominance, dualism began to pervade medical thinking. The mind was sundered from the body and seemed a thing apart, a spiritual rather than a scientific entity . . . To date, there is no methodology that objectifies perturbed inner states expressed by feelings of anxiety, tension, inadequacy, and depression. These emotional states are risk factors for illness, shaping the presentation of sickness, determining its progression and the speed of recovery. (p. 29-30)

When psychological problems dominate an illness, as is commonly the case, the general physician often diagnoses psychoneurosis, a wastebasket term to which are consigned a host of conditions lacking scientific explanations.

> The patient is seriously shortchanged by this dismissal of the psychological aspects of illness, and ignoring the emotional dimension lessens a doctor's capacity to ameliorate a chronic disease. Drugs may improve some of the presenting symptoms for a time, but the underlying illness is not healed. Inattention to the psychological domain fractures medicine at its heart by divorcing curing from healing. This common practice has injured the image of physicians and considerably diminished their standing in society. (p. 30)

I consider Dr Lown as a pioneer of introducing psychology in cardiology practice. He established the role of psychological stress on the cardiovascular system.

> A physician committed to healing cannot focus exclusively on a patient's chief complaint and deceased organs but must attend to the stressful aspects of the patient's life as well. This alerts the patient that the doctor is interested in him or her as a person, not just in the immediate problem. The patient is then more willing to share intimate and painful matters, and the doctor is better able to assess how healing is to be accomplished . . .
>
> The stresses that may be operating are as numerous and diverse as life itself. Generally, the most critical areas arise from work or family conflicts. If these are ignored, a chronic disease cannot be effectively addressed., whatever its anatomic location. While treatment with drugs alone may be temporarily effective, an entirely new symptom frequently fixates on a different bodily part. The chase to cure the patient

> is seemingly endless and ultimately frustrating to both the patient and the doctor. (p. 90)
>
> Far too frequently, the family psychopathology is so deep-seated that a cure is impossible. Healing, though is never impossible. Even in insoluble cases, a doctor's caring helps mitigate the misery and makes life more tolerable. (p. 96)

Towards the end of the book, Dr Lown mentions a story he called a modern Hasidic Tale about one of his patients. A Hasidic is a member of an ultra-Orthodox Judaism sect emphasising emotional and spiritual expression and pious devotion. The story began in 1974. One of his patients, he mentioned as S.V., was a humble, middle-aged man, short in stature, broad-shouldered, and ruggedly put together from Sicily in Italy, who had his mitral and aortic valves replaced by a leading cardiac surgeon in London. Dr Lown writes about how young SV survived the holocaust but yet a bacterial infection damaged the heart valves, and how he selected Dr Lown to be his doctor and travelled to the US multiple times at a significant cost over extended hospital stays there over thirteen years. He died in 1987.

Dr Lown called him a *Lamedvvovnik*, the hidden saint in the Jewish faith. In hindsight, Dr Lown feels that this patient came to him to inspire him in his career by his mere presence.

> The tipping point for maintaining human life on this planet is thirty-six people practising the sacred art of loving kindness at any given moment . . . However, these need not be the same

> thirty-six people at each moment . . . people step into and out of the *Lamedvvovnik* role, and that at any given moment, thirty-six people are stepping in.
>
> The greatest figures of prophecy and sanctity step forth out of the darkest night. But for the most part, the formative stream of the mystical life remains invisible. Certainly, the most decisive turning points in world history are substantially co-determined by souls whom no history book ever mentions. And we will only find out about those souls to whom we owe the decisive turning points in our personal lives on the day when all that is hidden is revealed.[28]

The whole point of undercover saints is that they stay hidden. Dwelling among the ordinary rank and file, they preserve their saintliness only by remaining outside established religious institutions. We may build edifices of ecclesiastical authority and hierarchies of piety. Still, the tradition of the *lamedvovniks* teaches that a spiritual leader should be humble enough to recognise that any of his congregants may be more righteous than him. This story left a deep impression on me. I started seeing some of my patients who are engaged with me over a very long period and found some reason to visit me, as SV did for Dr Lown, even if they can be seen by any other doctor more conveniently and at a lower price. I was never arrogant, but I consciously treated everyone with respect in my later life.

---

28 https://www.vermontcatholic.org/uncategorized/hidden-saints-the-legend-of-the-lamed-vavniks/. Last accessed on March 16, 2024.

Two questions about modern medicine remain far from settled: whether medicine is an "art based on science" and whether the "science of medicine" is a pure one or merely applied science. In my five decades of medical practice, I have seen the element of science in it is full of uncertainty. What is accepted as "scientific" by one generation of doctors is discarded by medical practitioners of the next generation in the light of newer evidence. Also, the "art of medicine" has not lost its sheen because advancements in science have made present-day medicine more sophisticated, but because doctors get too busy to spend time with their patients. Dr Lown asks to rely on the art of human understanding to "amplify the insights provided by science."[29] I have adapted his words as my policy and my message to the young doctors.

> At present, scientific medicine, even in a narrower sense, lacks precise solutions to most chronic ailments such as arthritis, heart disease, neurodegenerative disorders, autoimmune disease, and most cancers. While the scientific phase is quickening, we have a long way to go before these major disorders are fully understood. In the absence of a cure, these diseases require management, usually over a lifetime. The only available medical approach is to assuage symptoms, to slow and where possible halt a downhill course, to help the patient maintain a positive outlook, and to prevent the disease from taking charge of his or her life. These goals can be achieved only when patient expectations are narrowly focused on the attainable.

29 Bernard Lown, *The Lost Art of Healing: Practicing Compassion in Medicine*, New Delhi: Hay House India, 2009.

> An exaggerated attitude toward the potential of medicine proves self-defeating. In this age of hype, patients come to expect the impossible. They are not readily satisfied with mere abatement of symptoms but frequently demand non-existent cures. Pretensions of the healthcare industry and the godly posturing of some doctors contribute to such unreasonable expectations. Theatrical illusions are promoted by an unwholesome dynamic between hyperbolic professional claims and the public's inflated hypes.
>
> Unreal expectations heighten dissatisfaction for many who find that their conditions are not diagnosable, yet in my experience, the vast majority of symptoms lack exact explanations. The medical community has partially resolved this problem by devising meaningless diagnosis labels that mask ignorance rather than illuminate an underlying cause. (p. 314)

This brings me to the burning question of Artificial intelligence (AI) and the Art of Healing. Can patient care be enriched in the Digital Age?

It is easy to imagine the potential of AI to help people around the world live healthier lives. Some already use AI to spot early signs of disease quickly. A long-standing friend and Chairman of LV Prasad Eye Institute, Dr Gulapalli Nageswara Rao, is already using a special kind of camera designed to capture images of the eyes and evaluate them with AI. He distinguishes between "impact AI" in medicine and "glamour AI," meaning products that garner tantalising headlines but do not yet show hard evidence of patient benefit. Can there be a "caring AI" to retrieve the lost art of healing?

As I understand it, three dimensions of 'intelligence' operate in a doctor's work—physical, mental, and emotional. We can see surgical robots deployed there, operating with fantastic precision by integrating information technology and physical embodiment. Rather than replacing human surgeons, these machines generally require significant human supervision and interaction, meaning robotic surgery today is more accurately described as 'robot-assisted' surgery. Using increasingly sophisticated algorithms in robotics can facilitate more profound and more complex human-machine relationships with physical dimensions. The era of 'superstar' surgeons is already over, and one can see young surgeons doing great work with surgical robots.

Interpretive intelligence in radiology and pathology has also arrived, but as of 2024, it is still a work in progress. The algorithms still require large sets of high-quality training images annotated by human pathologists and programmers to learn how to diagnose a disease reliably and effectively. Applying machine learning algorithms in pathology can most accurately be described as 'machine-aided' or 'computer-assisted' pathology facilitating the emergence of algorithmically 'augmented pathologists.' There is currently no established way to explain why machine learning algorithms make a particular decision when interpreting digital slide images. With machines learning from every slide, I am curious to know if the interpretation of disease and its conceptualisation will change and the responses to it. Who will be held responsible and accountable for diagnostic errors?

The relationship between human subjectivity, the physiological affect, and algorithmic design works both ways: algorithms can also change how humans conceptualise, perceive, or effectively respond to the world, for example, by producing new categories of illness and disease from the data through identifying novel patterns of malignancy or correlations between population sub-groups and types of disease. Algorithmic activities, like profiling, re-ontologise the world by understanding and conceptualising it in new, unexpected ways and triggering and motivating actions based on the insights it generates.

This has important implications for medicine regarding how patients and illnesses are categorised and treated, including when new or emerging categories of infection or disease susceptibility align and in what manner. Irreversibly, digital pathology has challenged what has conventionally been largely a qualitative assessment of tissue samples by a human pathologist into an increasingly quantitative assessment co-performed by algorithms. Will it change the pathologists' embodied perception of diagnostics?

It is thus crucial to analyse how these technologies are transforming healthcare practices and to critically interrogate the meaning and nature of 'fair,' 'inclusive,' 'transparent' and 'accountable' analysis algorithms. I have concerns about fairness, transparency, bias, and accountability concerning algorithmic medicine. Who is behind all this development? Doctors? I am afraid not. How the shift to digital pathology alters the relational aspects of health and care practices is anyone's guess.

Will robotics in care delivery flourish in the face of shortages of healthcare personnel, ageing populations, and calls for improved quality of care? In combination with assistive physical technologies, developments in AI are currently facilitating the production of Socially Assistive Robots (SARs). These emotionally perceptive or intelligent machines represent a new site of affective relationality in care, designed to interact with humans via a communicative range that includes 'emotional' responses like interaction, communication, companionship, and moral support.

Narratives of intimacy, conventionally found in human relationships, are already being reproduced and embodied in interactions with humanoid robots. The robot's heart (*Kokoro* in Japanese language) emerges in the grey area between technological material and human imagination. Through tinkering and spectating, both robot builders and 'robot watchers' can experience the intimacy that results from apprehending the robot's heart. This experience creates an endless hermeneutic circle, drawing together subject and object, original and copy, creator and created, and watcher and watched to reconfigure participants' senses of their own *Kokoro*.

AI and robotics are already a part of our healthcare ecosystem, actively transforming the relationship between humans and machines in new affective, embodied, and relational ways. In addition to surgery, social robots have the potential to revolutionise care for ageing populations, helping people remain independent for longer and reducing the need for hospitalisation and care homes.

Besides, the use of these technologies also pertains to how different kinds of capabilities, skills and forms of 'intelligence' are being modelled into human-interfacing AI and robotic systems. There is an urgent need, or can I say a crying need, for doctors to participate in the development of the conceptual, normative, and ethical tools to understand and evaluate both AI-driven technologies and the changes they are making in the expression and manifestations of the affective and relational aspects of human experience. If medicine becomes a black box, it would be the saddest day for humanity and perhaps the first of the era that will lead it to its eventual extinction.

Bringing the art of healing back into medicine involves reemphasising healthcare's humanistic and compassionate aspects to complement the advances in science and technology. Doctors and nurses must prioritise empathetic communication, active listening, and patient-centred care to establish trust, build rapport, and create meaningful patient connections. Training programs can emphasise the importance of empathy in understanding patients' perspectives, concerns, and emotional needs. The involvement of senior practitioners in conducting such courses would be of great value and help.

We have practised a holistic approach to patient care that addresses not only the physical aspects of illness but also the emotional, social, and spiritual dimensions. A doctor must consider the whole person in their treatment plans, incorporating lifestyle factors, mental health support, and patient preferences into care decisions. Good doctors are known for the stories they share with their patients. Using narratives, storytelling, and reflective practices by the doctors deepens understanding, empathises with patient experiences, and fosters connection. Listening to the stories of patients behind their illnesses helps a doctor to understand patients' perspectives and learn the complexities of the human experience in healing.

Enhancing medicine's healing potential involves creating a hospital environment that does not resemble a laboratory or a hotel but prioritises the mind-body connection, patient-provider relationship, and healing environment. Create healing environments within healthcare settings that are calming, welcoming, and supportive of well-being. Natural light plays a critical role, and ideally, patients must be able to see the sky. A supportive and trusting environment can always be created where patients feel heard, understood, and valued. Communication that conveys warmth, understanding, and respect to enhance the healing process is always possible.

What is an ideal hospital environment for patients, providing the right conditions for something good to happen or exist? A conducive hospital environment is characterised by several key factors that promote healing, comfort, and overall well-being—cleanliness and hygiene, comfortable facilities, a quiet and peaceful atmosphere, and warm and caring staff—these are fundamental.

A good hospital must have a patient-centred design. Layouts prioritising easy access to care, clear signage, and spaces for family members can improve the overall experience for patients and visitors. Views of gardens or outdoor areas, as well as the incorporation of natural elements, can reduce stress and promote healing. Ensuring patient privacy through design (like private rooms or partitions) helps patients feel secure and respected. Providing nutritionally balanced meals and accommodating dietary needs can improve patient satisfaction, and health outcomes are equally important.

Perhaps the most neglected part, or absent aspect, is support services. Access to mental health resources, social workers, and patient advocates can help address emotional and social aspects of health. Involving patients in their care plans and decision-making fosters a sense of control and empowerment. Hospitals can create environments that significantly enhance the patient experience and support effective healing by focusing on these aspects.

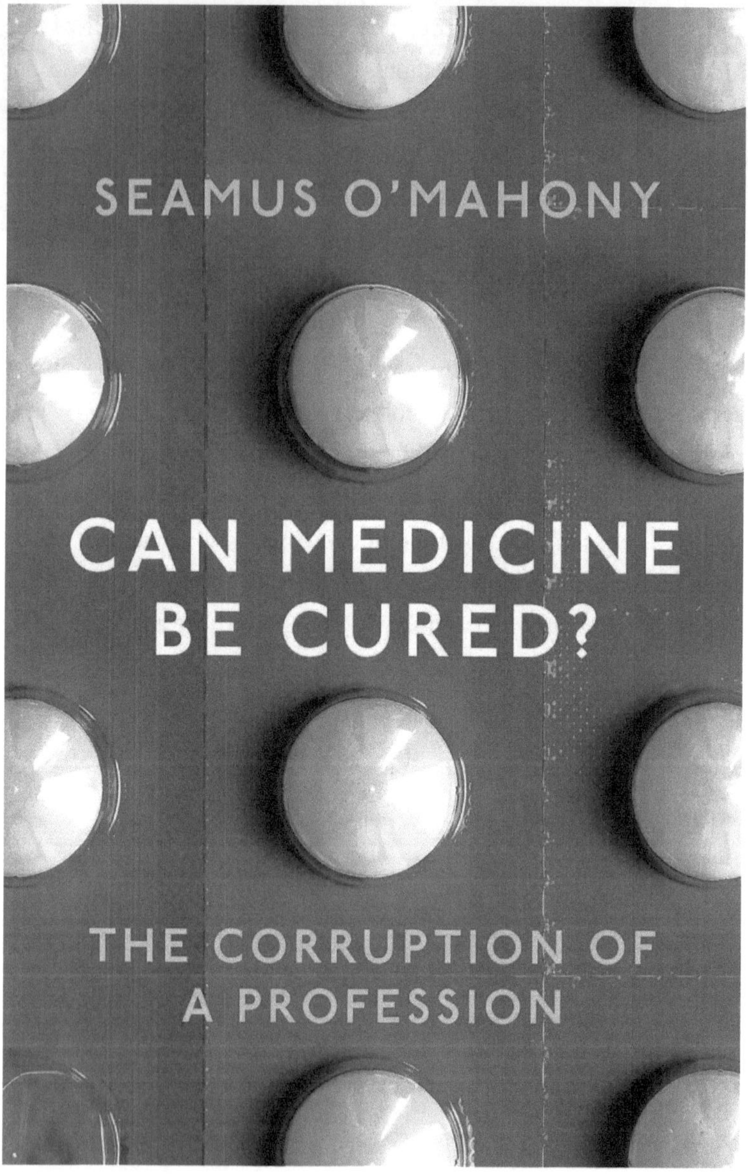
SEAMUS O'MAHONY
CAN MEDICINE BE CURED?
THE CORRUPTION OF A PROFESSION

Chapter 8

Practicing Right Medicine

So far in this book, starting with Hippocrates, I have attempted to present the evolution of medicine as a profession. It is no longer about one doctor treating a patient; it is a tradition - grooming young people to carry forward specific knowledge and skills accumulated by those who lived and practised it in the past - holding the baton from the earlier runner, run one's part of the sprint and then transfer it to the next runner in waiting. But what about the track? What if we are running on a treadmill? Is the medical profession's progress real, or is it all about doing more without adding value? There is a perception that medicine is more of a commerce now. Is it true? And if maladies crept into the profession, can they be cured?

Medicine has undergone significant changes in the new millennium, driven by technological advancements, which are dramatic in many aspects, especially diagnostics. Then, there are shifts in healthcare policy, notably the entry of government-provided medical insurance to every citizen. With such advancements, patient expectations will be transformed, and broader societal trends will follow. Improved diagnostic tools, minimally invasive surgical techniques, telemedicine, electronic health records (EHRs), and wearable health monitoring devices have arrived. These technologies have undoubtedly enhanced the accuracy and efficiency of medical diagnoses and treatments, but that is one side of the story.

Medicine has become overly reliant on advanced technologies and pharmaceuticals, often prioritising these interventions over more holistic approaches to health and wellness. There are concerns about the influence of financial interests, including pharmaceutical companies and for-profit healthcare institutions, on medical practice. This influence has already led to overprescribing of medications, unnecessary procedures, and a focus on profit rather than patient well-being. Socioeconomic status, race, ethnicity, and geographic location affect health conditions and treatment outcomes.

The rapid pace of medical advancement has also raised various ethical and legal challenges, such as patient privacy, data security, informed consent, end-of-life care, and emerging technologies such as gene editing, which are primarily experimental but available to those who can afford it. These developments necessitated systemic changes, including reforms in healthcare policy, medical education, and healthcare delivery models. The issue of the medical industry prioritising patient-centred care, equity, and ethical practice has become a complex one. While we cannot close doors to innovation, we cannot become a clinical trial hub either.

There are concerns about the influence of financial interests on healthcare delivery. Sometimes, healthcare organisations may be owned or heavily funded by private investors or corporations whose primary motivation is monetary profit. This can lead to decisions that prioritise financial gains over patient care, potentially resulting in practices such as overutilisation of medical services, unnecessary procedures, and high costs for patients. Furthermore, the rise of for-profit healthcare institutions and the increasing involvement of private equity firms in healthcare mergers and acquisitions have raised questions about the impact on the quality, accessibility, and affordability of healthcare services.

Seamus O'Mahony is an Irish gastroenterologist known for his contributions to medical literature and critical analyses of the healthcare system. Intrigued by its provocative title, *Can Medicine Be Cured?*[30] I read his book, which was published in 2019. Dr O'Mahony argues that medicine has become overly reliant on technology and pharmaceuticals, dehumanising patient care. He highlights the growing emphasis on treating symptoms rather than addressing underlying causes and the influence of financial interests on medical practice.

The book derives its credentials from its author, a doctor who has worked for many years in the NHS in the UK. This book is his second, after *The Way We Die*, published in 2017. It calls for reevaluating the current medical paradigm and advocating

30 Seamus O'Mahony, *Can Medicine Be Cured?*, London: Head of Zeus Ltd, 2019.

for a more holistic approach that prioritises the doctor-patient relationship and considers the social and environmental factors impacting health. I cannot entirely agree with Dr O'Mahony on every account. Still, his observations are well articulated and provide a 'ringside' view of the problems the medical profession faces in the modern era. I share his anxieties and cite some brilliantly written passages here.

> Since the 1980s, medical research has become a global business and driver of economies; it is the intellectual motor of the medical-industrial complex. It is seen by the public as a worthy philanthropic endeavour, carried out by altruists motivated only by a thirst for truth and a passion to cure disease and save lives . . . The great majority of medical research is a waste of time and money . . . (it) serves mainly the needs of the researchers and allied commercial interests. (p. 13-14)

Medical research has evolved into a global business and big money. Medical research increasingly involves collaboration among scientists, institutions, and pharmaceutical companies worldwide, demanding the pooling of resources, expertise, and data to capture the size of the modern healthcare industry, including pharmaceuticals, biotechnology, medical devices, and healthcare services, catering to the global market. The economic potential of investing in medical research and development to create innovative products and treatments that can be sold worldwide is the driving factor. Governments allocate significant funding to support research institutions and initiatives, while pharmaceutical companies and investors pour resources into drug discovery, clinical trials, and product development.

Cutting-edge medical research and technology attract patients worldwide seeking advanced treatments and procedures. Health tourism has become a booming industry in many countries, generating revenue from medical services, accommodations, and related expenses. Medical research creates jobs across various fields, including scientific research, clinical trials, regulatory affairs, manufacturing, sales, and marketing. These jobs contribute to economic growth, stability, and prosperity in communities where research facilities and pharmaceutical companies are located. For these reasons, medical research has become integral to the global economy, driving innovation, creating jobs, and improving healthcare outcomes worldwide. It has become too big to be controlled by any government.

> There is a philosophical, moral, and existential paradox at the heart of research. Death is the inevitable product of disease, ageing and the body's breakdown. Research aims to 'fight' this, yet we accept, deep within our being, that death is not only inevitable, it is *good* . . . The dramatic increase in human longevity witnessed in the twentieth century is so new and so dramatic that, as a species, we haven't learned how to deal with it. (p. 50)

Even when death is inevitable, research aimed at prolonging life serves several vital purposes. Rather than fatal, cancers are increasingly turning into chronic diseases. Treatments and interventions can alleviate symptoms, manage pain, and enhance comfort, allowing individuals to live their remaining time with dignity and as much independence as possible. But even more than that, studies aimed at prolonging life contribute to our understanding of disease mechanisms, treatment strategies, and the human body's resilience. Even if specific interventions do not ultimately extend life expectancy, they can yield valuable insights that inform future research and benefit patients with similar conditions.

Additionally, advances in medical research can stimulate innovation, drive economic growth, and create employment opportunities in healthcare and related industries. After all, education, effort, scientific development, and technological advancement cannot be achieved with a nihilist mindset. While death is an inevitable part of the human experience, research aimed at prolonging life reflects our collective efforts to alleviate suffering, provide hope, and promote human flourishing, even in the face of life-limiting illnesses.

> Medicine is an applied science, not a pure science. Many would say that it is not a science at all; it is a craft and practice. In many ways, science and medicine are antithetical: doubt is at the very core of science, but doctors who express doubt are not highly regarded by their patients. This reflects the contemporary combination of consumerism in health care and the Cartesian belief that our bodies are machines and should be mended as efficiently and unfussily as a broken kitchen appliance. (p. 98)

So, what defines the right medicine in these times? There are limits to technology when it is not used correctly or when it is used to replace people completely. The main job of healthcare workers in hospitals, nursing homes, and other places is to take care of patients. They need technology to help those workers do their jobs. Clinicians do not need technology that derails their work. While finding, understanding, and reporting treatments' positive effects has become more accessible, making progress in finding, interpreting, and reporting their adverse effects has become more demanding. It is also easy to mix up side effects with the signs of the illness being treated. People who take painkillers for headaches may get headaches caused by the painkillers, for example.

Pharmaceutical companies develop, manufacture, and market drugs and medications for various health conditions. They invest heavily in R&D to discover new medicines and treatments. The medical technology sector is another engine of progress. It produces medical imaging systems, surgical instruments, prosthetics, and implantable devices. Hospitals, clinics, and healthcare providers offer specialised treatments and surgeries. The situation gets complicated after health insurance companies and managed care organisations are intensified. While hospitals aim at more revenue from every bed, these entities operate to minimise the costs of treating the insured patient.

However, the most significant impact has yet to arrive in the era of biotechnology. A vibrant biotechnology industry is developing products and technologies derived from biological systems, such as therapeutic proteins, gene therapies, and biopharmaceuticals.

These hold immense promise for transforming medicine in the coming years. Advances in genomic sequencing, biomarker identification, and data analytics allow for more precise diagnosis, prognosis, and treatment selection across various diseases, including cancer, rare genetic disorders, and chronic conditions. Biotechnology will undoubtedly revolutionise medicine in the next few years by offering innovative therapies, enhancing diagnostic capabilities, and ushering in a new era of personalised and precision medicine.

Reflecting on how medicine has evolved in my lifetime, I can see that multidisciplinary teams have replaced the doctor. Such teams include healthcare professionals from various specialities, including doctors, nurses, pharmacists, social workers, physical therapists, and more. This diversity allows for comprehensive care, simultaneously addressing multiple aspects of a patient's health. The "clinical aristocrats" and "god-like" doctors that we have seen earlier, who possess absolute authority and knowledge in medical decision-making, are now extinct. Dr O'Mahony writes:

> Following the collapse of the power of the clinical-aristocrats, the vacuum was filled by managers and a new breed called clinical directors, who viewed their roles through a managerial prism . . . Power within medicine seeped out of the hospitals to the committee rooms and the universities . . . the committee men and women sought prestige in the royal colleges, professional bodies, and medical schools. Clinical work was strictly for the unambitious. All of this has left the hospitals essentially leaderless. Managers and clinical directors are nominally in charge, but they are motivated

> mainly by targets and metrics and are unconcerned with maintaining the 'invisible glue' which once held hospitals together. (p. 195)

While there has been a shift from paternalistic models of medicine towards more patient-centred and collaborative approaches, it would be inaccurate to declare the end of the era of god-like doctors outright. Instead, there has been a transition towards a more balanced and equitable relationship between patients and healthcare providers, characterised by mutual respect, shared decision-making, and transparency.

Several factors have contributed to this evolution. Thanks to the Internet, patients today are more informed than ever before. They actively participate in healthcare decisions, ask questions, and seek second opinions. This promotes critical thinking, scientific inquiry, and the use of clinical guidelines to guide medical practice, reducing reliance on individual physician authority or intuition. And yet, doctors remain highly respected and trusted figures, valued for their expertise, compassion, and dedication to patient care. The evolving role of doctors emphasises collaboration, empathy, and communication skills, fostering partnerships with patients based on trust, respect, and shared decision-making. Ultimately, the transformation of the doctor-patient relationship reflects broader changes in healthcare culture, ethics, and values towards a more patient-centered and equitable approach to care.

> Medicine no longer knows what it is *for*. Is the ultimate aim of medical research to eliminate all disease? If so, then it must be aiming, too to make us immortal? Even if that were

> possible (which it isn't), are we quite sure that we want it? Is the aim of clinical medicine now to keep the entire adult population under permanent surveillance by screening for an increasing number of diseases? Does longevity trump all other considerations? (p. 265)

The intersection of digital health and surveillance raises important questions about privacy, data security, and ethical considerations. While digital health technologies offer numerous benefits for individuals and healthcare systems, there are concerns about the potential for surveillance and misuse of personal health data. Digital health technologies, such as wearable devices, mobile health apps, and remote monitoring tools, collect vast amounts of personal health data, including biometric information, medical history, and lifestyle habits. However, collecting and storing sensitive health information raises privacy risks for individuals, as unauthorised access or data breaches could compromise confidentiality and expose personal details. Additionally, aggregating and analysing health data across populations could lead to identifying individuals or groups and their "branding".

In some contexts, digital health technologies may be used for surveillance purposes by governments, employers, insurers, or other entities to monitor individuals' health behaviours, adherence to medical treatments, or compliance with public health guidelines. This surveillance could infringe on individuals' autonomy, freedom of movement, and privacy rights. Using digital health data for surveillance raises ethical questions about autonomy, consent, and the balance between public health interests and individual rights. There are concerns about the potential for discrimination, stigmatisation, and unequal access to healthcare services based on individuals' health data or risk profiles.

Transparency and accountability are essential for addressing concerns about surveillance in digital health. Clear policies, informed consent processes, and robust security measures are needed to safeguard individuals' privacy and trust in digital health technologies. Additionally, oversight, audit, and recourse mechanisms should be in place to hold accountable those responsible for data misuse or breaches. We must not create a modern Frankenstein. While digital health technologies offer transformative potential for improving healthcare delivery and outcomes, addressing concerns about surveillance, privacy, and ethical implications is crucial. By prioritising transparency, data security, and individual rights, stakeholders can harness the benefits of digital health while mitigating risks and safeguarding privacy in an increasingly connected healthcare landscape.

Can the modern healthcare industry be called a "mendacity," as Dr O'Mahony fears it to become? The term "mendacity" typically refers to deceitfulness or dishonesty, suggesting that there may be elements within the industry that are not transparent or truthful. My answer is a firm "No". Every doctor must resist trends toward this at every level of their work. While the healthcare industry undoubtedly faces challenges and criticisms, it is essential to acknowledge that it also plays a crucial role in promoting public health, treating illness, and advancing medical science. However, like any complex system, it is not without its flaws. Healthcare costs are high, and access to efficient care is limited for affluent people, leading to disparities in health outcomes. The pursuit of profit in corporation-run hospitals fundamentally conflicts with the delivery of optimal patient care. Overusing medical interventions, inappropriate prescribing practices, and unnecessary procedures have become an order of the day.

Reducing errors through better training, technology, and systems, ensuring all populations have access to high-quality healthcare., making healthcare more affordable and reducing financial barriers, and enhancing the focus on patient needs, preferences, and values are "musts" and there can be no slack in any one of these areas, whether all diseases can be cured, the answer is more complex. Many diseases can be cured with current medical knowledge, such as bacterial infections with antibiotics, certain cancers with surgery, radiation, and chemotherapy, and some chronic diseases with advanced treatments.

However, diseases, such as certain genetic disorders, chronic conditions, and viral infections like HIV, currently have no cure but can often be managed with ongoing treatment. Ongoing research continues to progress in finding cures for more diseases, including advancements in gene therapy, immunotherapy, and personalised medicine. From a philosophical perspective, addressing systemic issues such as health inequities, ethical practices, and holistic health can be called "cures". Who can deny the importance of reducing disparities in health outcomes among different populations, ensuring ethical standards are upheld in medical research and practice and promoting a holistic approach to health that includes physical, mental, and social well-being?

Can medicine be cured? It is asking the wrong question. Medicine is a dynamic and continually advancing discipline that improves human health and well-being. Medicine adapts and evolves in response to discoveries, emerging diseases, and changing health challenges. There is a cloud of questions that need answers. Can urbanisation be stopped? Can the rampant proliferation of industrially processed foods reign? Can health prevention be made a part of education and HR policy? Can people be encouraged to live simple and balanced lives? Can nutritional security be provided to all sections of society, especially children and the poor? And if the answer is no, then why single out the medical profession, the healthcare industry, and especially the doctors for a misplaced reprimand and browbeating?

There are no quick fixes. It is an ongoing journey of discovery, improvement, and adaptation. While individual diseases and medical practices can be improved and sometimes eradicated, the field of medicine itself is a dynamic and evolving science dedicated to understanding and enhancing human health. The goal is continuous improvement, innovation, and addressing the multifaceted challenges that arise in healthcare. Every successive generation of doctors needs to capture the spirit of 'not harm the patient', embrace what is new on offer, and improve the 'practice' as medicine is rightly called a profession. This is what I call the right medicine.

Undoubtedly, the medical profession, as a crucial pillar of society, has reoriented its priorities to address the challenges of increasing life expectancy and societal consumerism. However, the extent to which this shift has led to the neglect of vital aspects such as emergency rooms, general surgery operation theatres, and community clinics varies across countries. In the context of India, it stands between Cuba and the USA, with no discernible impact to change on all fronts. Unlike compassion and professionalism, this impact is not easily quantifiable, which unfortunately allows managers, politicians, and even our patients to perceive doctors as if in an eclipse.

Dr O'Mahony talked about what he thought were the seemingly impossible problems in modern medicine. He pointed out that Big Pharma had led to the pointless growth of academic and research medicine. Imprudent, pricey projects like the Human Genome Project bother him, and it is a fact that so far, we have yet to see many benefits compared to the money and time spent on them. Dr O'Mahony seconds Dr Major Greenwood, an epidemiologist and statistician who wrote in the 1930s that modern medicine may be unable to "cure all disease" or "defeat cancer." Still, it can try to "make the condition of human life everywhere more bearable."

I often think about whether I would have chosen to be a doctor if I knew what I know now about the state of medicine 60 years ago. The answer is still yes for me, but I know it could be very different for the next group of doctors. Low morale among good young doctors is a significant problem; we are not dealing with it quickly enough.

In the movie "The Last Czars," Emperor Nicholas asks his communist attackers why they put him in jail when he loves and is loyal to Russia. The revolutionaries say, "You loved Russia, but not the Russians." So, love your patients as much as you love your careers, if not more. To help medical students understand how medicine and culture work today, I try to get them to spend more time with the arts and humanities.

Studying the arts and humanities improves doctors' communication with patients and their families. This includes understanding nonverbal cues, fostering empathy, and building rapport, which is essential in clinical settings. A background in the humanities encourages a more holistic view of patients, seeing them as individuals with emotions, experiences, and social contexts rather than just medical cases. This approach promotes better understanding and more personalised care. The arts and humanities stimulate critical thinking, analytical skills, and creativity. These skills are essential in medical practice for diagnosing complex cases and thinking outside the box when developing treatment plans.

Engagement with literature, philosophy, and the arts plays a significant role in cultivating empathy. Medical professionals who appreciate human experiences and narratives can better relate to patients' challenges, leading to more compassionate care. It also serves as a form of stress relief, helping doctors to counteract the emotional toll of their work and supporting their mental health. By blending medical training with insights and skills from the arts and humanities, doctors can enhance their practice and provide more effective, empathetic, and comprehensive patient care. Overall, the medical humanities strive to strengthen the practice of medicine by promoting a more holistic approach to healthcare that values the human experience alongside scientific knowledge.

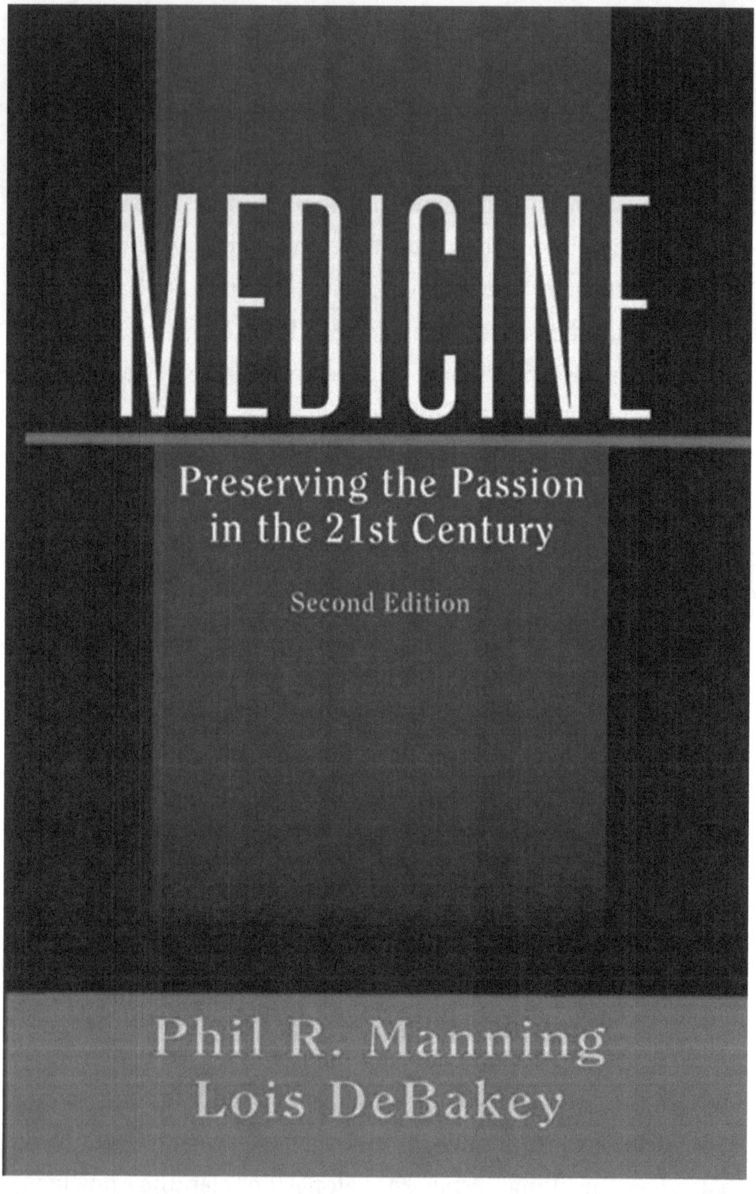
MEDICINE
Preserving the Passion
in the 21st Century
Second Edition
Phil R. Manning
Lois DeBakey

Chapter 9
Preserving the Passion

As has been my habit and advice to my colleagues and students, reading good books is integral to a medical doctor's life. Reading books, mainly written by great doctors or about them, instils pride and commitment by supporting continuous learning, clinical excellence, critical thinking, empathy, professional development, well-being, and personal growth. By embracing the habit of reading, doctors can enhance their practice, enrich their lives, and make meaningful contributions to the healthcare profession and the well-being of their patients. I consider *Medicine: Preserving the Passion in the 21st Century* by Phil R. Manning and Lois DeBakey a must-read for medical doctors.

In its purest sense, a profession is a paid job that requires extensive training and formal qualifications. Passion on the other hand means a strong desire that drives you to learn and do more.

Dr Manning offers insights into maintaining passion and purpose in medicine in this thought-provoking book. It resonated well with my style of storytelling and indulging in literature and the arts to foster empathy, reflection, and self-awareness. This is the best way for healthcare professionals to enhance their ability to provide compassionate and patient-centred care and, more importantly, avert despair and burnout.

The book, co-authored by Lois DeBakey, professor of scientific communications at Baylor College of Medicine, is a collage of writings by leading medical professionals. It explores medicine's rich history, tracing its evolution from ancient healing practices to modern healthcare. Practitioners highlight the timeless values and principles that have guided them in their careers, emphasising the importance of compassion, integrity, and the doctor-patient relationship. It offers perhaps the most authentic view of the complex challenges confronting healthcare professionals in the 21st century, covering various aspects such as technological advancements, bureaucratic pressures, and ethical dilemmas. It discusses the impact of healthcare reform, managed care, and regulatory changes on the practice of medicine, as well as the growing prevalence of burnout and disillusionment among physicians.

The book derives its value from the insights from the medical fraternity across the United States into how healthcare professionals can preserve their passion and sense of purpose in adversity. The importance of self-care, resilience, and maintaining a strong sense of professional identity amidst the demands of modern healthcare practice can never be ignored. I could relate well to the small articles written by various doctors. I picked a few passages to address important topics concerning medical doctors when they work as interns and residents and later join hospitals or practice in clinics.

> Some physicians fail to become immersed in their practice because they allow it to become too routine. This is primarily an attitudinal problem, for almost any practice environment can be made stimulating . . . My teacher . . . used to admonish us that each clinical case is a research project . . . look for the unanswered research questions in every routine issue. The rewards have been ample. In just the past year, 'routine' cases uncovered interesting information. A depressed patient with porphyria led to a literature review and the discovery that porphyric psychosis is omitted from the current textbook of medicine; a case of pseudo-seizure led to the demonstration of a basic linkage in the thought-speech process; a case of self-mutilation led to the description of a new clinical syndrome; a case of dissociation led to the analysis of visceral brain components of consciousness . . . surely enough excitement in one year to keep a jaded administrator alive and enthusiastically on his toes to see what the next 'routine case' will turn up. (p. 13)

Overall, both clinic settings and large hospitals offer valuable learning experiences for doctors. Doctors learn in various ways, depending on whether they work in clinics or join large hospitals. There are some key differences, and it is vital to know them while making a choice that will mainly become a lifetime decision.

> Paul White [American physician and cardiologist (1886 –1973)] used to say that the excitement of medicine had to do with the fact that medicine could link science to humanism. He was a kind, gentle man who did not urge, cajole, or plead

> with people to perform, but because of his own stand of excellence, he inspired others to achieve . . .
>
> He defined a complete diagnosis as one including aetiology, altered anatomy, altered physiology, and functional cardiac status---a classification later adopted by the New York Heart Association. He was also a prophet. He predicted the role of "risk factors" in cases of coronary atherosclerosis disease and taught how to prevent the disease in the later 1940s . . . He used to say that a trainee should see patient one-third of the day, teach one-third of the day, and write one-third of the day. (p. 44-45)

Dr White was pivotal in advancing the understanding and treatment of cardiovascular diseases. He was instrumental in popularising the use of the electrocardiogram (ECG) in clinical practice and recognised its diagnostic value in assessing various cardiac conditions, including arrhythmias and myocardial infarction. He researched heart disease extensively, particularly the relationship between diet, exercise, and heart health. His studies contributed to understanding preventive cardiology and lifestyle interventions for cardiovascular disease prevention. He championed initiatives such as smoking cessation, regular exercise, and a heart-healthy diet.

Heart disease is often multifactorial, meaning that multiple risk factors can contribute to its development, but I must mention that one of the most significant risk factor for heart disease is hypertension. High blood pressure puts strain on the heart and blood vessels, leading to atherosclerosis – arteries getting hardened and narrowed - which can increase the risk of heart attack, stroke, and other cardiovascular complications. Other significant risk factors for heart disease include elevated levels of LDL cholesterol, inhaling harmful chemicals during smoking that can damage the heart and blood vessels, increasing the risk of heart disease, heart attack, stroke, diabetes, and other metabolic abnormalities. The pathogenesis of atherosclerosis remains a research topic and preventing it is the only way out.

Regular exercise, maintaining a healthy weight, eating a balanced diet, not smoking, managing stress, and controlling hypertension, diabetes, and high cholesterol are all crucial steps in preventing heart disease. Obesity, especially the waistline type, must not be ignored and attended to. The inflammatory substances released by visceral fat promote inflammation throughout the body, including within the arteries. Chronic inflammation contributes to endothelial dysfunction, which is a precursor to atherosclerosis.

> Every physician, whether a specialist or a general internist, should select some clinical condition and begin, at an early date, to develop special knowledge and experience about its natural course and its diagnostic and therapeutic management. Systemic lupus erythematosus, bacterial endocarditis, and giant-cell arteries, for example, have intrigued me through the years, always as a result of my having seen a patient with the condition. Seeing the patient was followed by a gathering of articles, compilation of filing index, and slow, methodical collection of case material.

> Developing subjects of special interest has several advantages. First, it keeps the clinician intellectually stimulated instead of submerged in the purely routine. Second, in examining the natural history of a disease over time, the physician will acquire a richer knowledge of many other disorders that may simulate it. Third, such clinical studies, if carried out well, may lead to a clinical report, and such a report sometimes leads to an important advance in medicine. Finally, from a purely practical standpoint, such studies help the young clinician becoming established as a consultant . . .
>
> Clinicians, then, should be permanent, enthusiastic students of disease and of human beings affected by it so that they may acquire the ability to cure illness or relieve discomfort and to afford compassion and support to their patients. Without a practical and vital program of continued self-education, these priest-like powers of the superior clinician cannot be fully realized. (p. 87-88)

Clinical cardiologists typically work closely with patients to assess risk factors, perform diagnostic tests, develop treatment plans, and provide ongoing medical management, including medication prescriptions and lifestyle management. Interventional cardiologists, on the other hand, specialise in performing minimally invasive procedures to diagnose and treat cardiovascular conditions, particularly those involving the coronary arteries and structural heart defects. They are trained to perform interventions - cardiac catheterisation procedures - such as angioplasty and stent placement to open blocked arteries and restore blood flow to the heart and repair heart valves, close congenital defects, or manage other complex cardiac conditions using catheter-based techniques.

It is essential to recognise that clinical and interventional cardiologists undergo extensive training and possess specialised skills necessary for comprehensive cardiovascular care. The choice between pursuing a career as a clinical cardiologist or an interventional cardiologist often depends on individual interests, aptitudes, and career aspirations. Some cardiologists may focus exclusively on clinical practice, while others may pursue additional training in interventional cardiology to perform procedures and interventions. Rather than comparing the superiority of clinical versus interventional cardiologists, it is more appropriate to recognise the complementary roles they play within the broader field of cardiovascular medicine. Both specialities contribute valuable expertise to improving patient outcomes and advancing the treatment of cardiovascular disease.

> The common thread through all of academic life is teaching, and although academicians may develop individual styles, anyone can learn to be an effective teacher if the desire to impart knowledge is sincere and if sufficient time and effort are invested . . . An effective teacher cares about students as people beyond their training . . . The ideal teacher is enthusiastic, has a good sense of humour, sets standards that motivate students to do their best, and has a broad knowledge base organised in a way that the trainee readily understands. (p. 256)

> A common mistake made by those in medical education . . . is assuming that events such as graduation from medical school and completion of residency or fellowship mark the end of something. In reality, they mark the beginning of a career of perpetual study. The recent graduate should be prepared for his clinical training program, and the finishing resident should be prepared for his lifelong study. By this time, the habit of critical reading should have been established, as well as the self-evaluation and honest self-criticism that are essential for continued intellectual growth and maintenance of clinical skills. The source of useful knowledge and information for physicians is often self-instruction. (p. 258)

I loved teaching, and students somehow found me even in my corporate hospital career. What attracted them to my way of teaching? What was it that I was sharing with them the knowledge that their professors in the medical school had not? A few of my students, after becoming accomplished doctors in various specialities, some of them cardiologists, told me they loved my discussions on one of the biggest mysteries in cardiology - the onset of atherosclerosis. The exact triggers that initiate the development of atherosclerosis in seemingly healthy arteries have yet to be fully understood, even now in the 2020s. Various factors, such as endothelial dysfunction, inflammation, oxidative stress, and lipid abnormalities, are believed to contribute to the initiation of plaque formation. Earlier thought of as a dull fat storage disease, it is now seen as an ongoing inflammatory response.

Still, the precise sequence of events remains a mystery. Unlocking the secrets of atherosclerosis could lead to developing more targeted and personalised approaches for preventing and treating cardiovascular disease, ultimately improving outcomes for millions of patients worldwide. I am unsure if I will see the unveiling of this mystery in my lifetime, but chronic inflammation within the arterial wall is a hallmark of atherosclerosis. I therefore tell my patients to have a healthy diet, exercise regularly, and quit smoking without any ifs and buts.

The general perception is that the concept of paternalistic doctors, whom patients consider benevolent figures, is over. However, I am frequented by the fourth generation of some of my early patients, who are full of faith. What they do not trust is the insurance system. Hospital managers are both dreaded and scorned.

> The hard fact is that over the years most of us did become complacent. Many lost some sensitivity . . . We also suffered a lapse of intellectual discipline. In our naïve zeal to 'leave no stone unturned' on behalf of our patients, we neglected the realities of fiscal responsibility. In our benignly paternalistic fashion, we did things our way for a long time. And this is how the unwelcome nose of the managed care camel succeeded in creeping under our tent. Undoubtedly, managed care has imposed a renewed sense of fiscal discipline on medicine. But as it exists, it has excessive warts. (p. 419)

While the paternalistic healthcare model is no longer considered ideal, there is recognition that the relationship between patients and healthcare providers should be one of collaboration and mutual respect, with patients playing an active role in their care. My message to young doctors is to continue to be paternalistic. While the era of paternalistic doctors may be diminishing, there are still situations where a more directive approach from doctors is necessary and appropriate. For example, in emergencies where patients may be unable to make decisions for themselves or when they cannot understand their medical condition or treatment options, doctors must act in the patient's best interests. Put your foot down, even if no one asks, and decide on behalf of the patient. Do not allow "managers" and "executives" to manipulate the family. Equally important is to stop the family from floating indecisively.

> If you approach the clinical puzzles in medical practice as intellectual challenges, if you acquire the habit of reading and discussing with colleagues and a steady flow of new medical information issuing from scientists and scholars, if you evaluate your clinical results regularly, framing precise questions and obtaining answers to the questions arising in practice; and if you view each patient not as a clinical case; but as a fellow human being whose unstated fears, anxieties, and dependence associated with illness also require attention, you will be rewarded with professional satisfaction and personal enjoyment, and you will assuredly preserve the passion for medicine that led you into this noble humanitarian profession. (p. 441)

I consider a medical doctor's passion an inward energy, intense enthusiasm, dedication, and commitment to medicine. It goes beyond mere interest or career choice and involves a strong emotional connection to medicine, the well-being of patients, and the pursuit of knowledge and excellence in healthcare. In terms of actions for such passionate doctors, I have articulated three hallmarks - desire to help others, commitment to lifelong learning, and resilience and dedication. I exclude the fashionable virtues of empathy and compassion, which I consider a fundamental quality of a human being and cannot be ascribed to the medical profession. In the rest of this chapter, I will elaborate on these three hallmarks of a passionate medical doctor.

The desire to help others is a fundamental aspect of being passionate about medicine and genuinely wanting to impact people's lives positively. For a modern doctor, the desire to help others encompasses a range of responsibilities and approaches that extend beyond traditional clinical practice. Modern doctors can prioritise patient-centred care, which involves understanding each patient's unique needs, preferences, and values. They should strive to build trusting relationships with patients, involve them in shared decision-making, and tailor treatments to individual circumstances. Modern doctors can advocate for their patients personally and on broader social and systemic healthcare issues. They may work to ensure equitable access to care, address social determinants of health, and promote policies that improve health outcomes for all.

Doctors can recognise the importance of preventive medicine in promoting overall health and reducing the burden of chronic diseases. They educate patients about healthy lifestyle choices, recommend screenings and vaccinations, and guide disease prevention and health promotion. Above all, wilful collaboration with other healthcare professionals in the interest of the patients, including other doctors, nurses, pharmacists, therapists, and social workers, is essential for modern doctors—the value of interdisciplinary teamwork in providing comprehensive and coordinated care to patients is immense. A passionate doctor of the 21st century must never shy away from educating patients and communities, engaging in global and public health initiatives, and practising ethically.

A doctor must commit to lifelong learning as medical knowledge and technology constantly evolve. New treatments, medications, diagnostic tools, and guidelines are developed regularly. Lifelong learning ensures that doctors stay updated with the latest evidence-based practices and are equipped to provide the best possible care to their patients. Doctors who engage in ongoing education are better equipped to diagnose conditions accurately, develop appropriate treatment plans, and manage complex cases effectively. Besides, lifelong learning enhances doctors' professional growth and development, refines their clinical skills, expands their areas of expertise, and helps them pursue specialised training or certifications in specific fields of medicine. Staying abreast of new developments in medical ethics and healthcare policies is also essential to navigating ethical dilemmas, upholding patient rights, and maintaining high standards of professionalism and integrity. Above all, continuous learning helps doctors identify and mitigate potential risks to patient safety. By staying updated on best practices, evidence-based guidelines, and patient safety initiatives, doctors can minimise errors, adverse events, and prevent patient harm. Lifelong learners are more likely to become leaders and innovators. By staying curious, exploring new ideas, and challenging existing paradigms, doctors can drive positive change, contribute to medical research, and shape the future of healthcare delivery.

Resilience coupled with dedication is a defining hallmark trait of a medical doctor. Modern doctors face numerous professional challenges, including long hours, high workload, complex cases, and emotional stress. Resilience enables them to bounce back from setbacks, cope with adversity, and continue providing quality care despite difficult circumstances. Doctors must remain steadfast in upholding ethical principles, such as patient autonomy, beneficence, non-maleficence, and justice, even in challenging situations. Resilient and dedicated doctors are more likely to embrace innovation and drive positive change in healthcare. They persist in exploring new treatment modalities, technologies, and approaches to improve patient outcomes and enhance care delivery. Overall, resilience and dedication are essential qualities that enable modern doctors to navigate the complexities of their profession, provide compassionate care to patients, advocate for their well-being, collaborate effectively with colleagues, uphold ethical standards, and drive innovation in healthcare.

While some may argue that modern doctors are more focused on their careers, it is essential to recognise that most medical professionals enter the field with a genuine desire to care for patients. However, the evolving landscape of healthcare, increasing administrative tasks, and financial pressures can sometimes shift the focus towards career advancement.

To ensure that caring for patients remains the primary focus, doctors can reconnect with their initial motivation for entering the medical field, prioritise patient-centred care and empathy in all interactions, maintain a healthy work-life balance to prevent burnout and advocate for changes in the healthcare system that prioritise patient care over profit. By consciously reflecting on their priorities and committing to patient well-being, doctors can balance their career ambitions and their passion for caring for patients.

Passion can indeed be perpetuating and sustaining over time. Passion serves as a powerful source of motivation. When individuals encounter difficulties or failures, their passion for their pursuits can provide the energy and determination to overcome barriers and keep moving forward. Passion is also contagious and can inspire others to share in one's enthusiasm. When individuals passionately pursue their goals and dreams, they often inspire those around them to do the same, creating a ripple effect of motivation and positivity. Based on experience, I can confidently tell you that self-care activities such as exercise, mindfulness, hobbies, and spending time with loved ones keep your passion alive and growing.

To enhance their passion for patient care, doctors must connect with patients on a deeper level. Only this helps them genuinely care for their well-being. Listening to patients without interruption can build trust and show genuine concern for their experiences and needs. Staying updated on medical advancements and new treatment options can ignite a doctor's passion for providing the best care possible. By spending more time with every patient in their practice, a doctor can reignite and strengthen their passion for patient care.

Taking care of oneself physically, mentally, and emotionally can prevent burnout and help a doctor maintain their enthusiasm for patient care. It was never easy, and it will be challenging. Surround yourself with like-minded individuals who share your passions. Engage in meaningful conversations, collaborate on projects, and build supportive relationships that nurture and sustain your enthusiasm. Above all, feel good that you are a doctor.

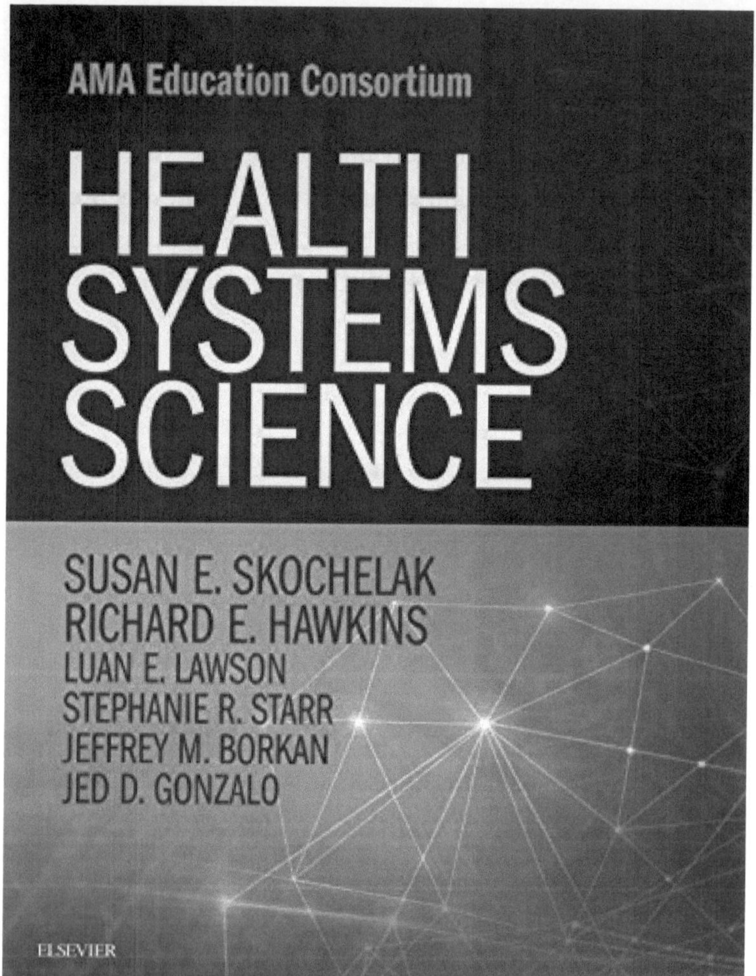
AMA Education Consortium
HEALTH
SYSTEMS
SCIENCE
SUSAN E. SKOCHELAK
RICHARD E. HAWKINS
LUAN E. LAWSON
STEPHANIE R. STARR
JEFFREY M. BORKAN
JED D. GONZALO
ELSEVIER

Chapter 10
Health Systems Science

As modern healthcare becomes organised and corporatised, it is not just about individual patient care but the systems and structures that support and deliver that care that decide the cost and quality of the outcomes. Health Systems Science (HSS) is an emerging interdisciplinary field that focuses on understanding and improving the complex systems involved in healthcare delivery. It encompasses various topics, including healthcare delivery models, quality improvement, patient safety, health policy, healthcare economics, healthcare technology, and population health.

As a formal field, HSS has had various initiators and has evolved due to contributions from multiple disciplines and individuals within healthcare, public health, health policy, and related fields. However, certain individuals and organisations have played significant roles in shaping and promoting the field. The work of American physician and health economist Dr David M. Eddy has contributed to the development of methods for evaluating the effectiveness and efficiency of healthcare interventions and delivery models.

The Institute of Medicine (IOM) in the United States has been instrumental in promoting research and education related to health systems and healthcare delivery. Through reports such as *Crossing the Quality Chasm: A New Health System for the 21st Century* and *To Err is Human: Building a Safer Health System*, the IOM has highlighted the importance of addressing system-level issues to improve healthcare quality and patient safety. For the first time, medicine is not only seen as a system – not art, not science, not a doctor-patient transaction, but a system wherein hundreds of people work together to serve patients. And it has been brought out that this system is prone to errors.

I cite three passages from these reports here to illustrate the reality of the workplace where doctors perform in the modern world. A huge system operates between them and their patients, and any error in that system may harm a patient, for which the doctor is held responsible, even if not legally punished but emotionally condemned and cursed.

> A healthcare system can be defined as a set of connected or interdependent parts or agents—including caregivers and patients—bound by a common purpose and acting on their knowledge. Health care is complex because of the great number of interconnections within and among small care systems. For example, office practices and critical care units in hospitals are linked to other units (such as laboratories and emergency departments) and are often embedded in even larger "umbrella" organizations such as hospitals, health plans, and integrated delivery systems.

> Healthcare systems are adaptive because unlike mechanical systems, they are composed of individuals—patients and clinicians who have the capacity to learn and change as a result of experience. Their actions in delivering health care are not always predictable, and tend to change both their local and larger environments. The unpredictability of behavior in complex adaptive systems can be seen as contributing to huge variations in the delivery of health care. If such a system is to improve its performance . . . some of these actions need to be specified to the extent possible so they are predictable with a high level of reliability.[31]

Healthcare delivery systems are incredibly complex, involving numerous interactions between providers, patients, technology, medications, and procedures. With so many variables at play, the potential for error increases. Being operated by humans systems are indeed susceptible to human errors.

> Organizations and clinicians that act as though they have nothing to hide become more trustworthy. The health care system should seek to earn renewed trust not by hiding its defects, but by revealing them, along with making a relentless commitment to improve. The transition to openness is a difficult one for our often-beleaguered health care organizations, but it is a journey worth making. In the longer run, access to information can inspire trust among patients and caregivers that the system is working effectively to advance

31 https://www.med.unc.edu/neurosurgery/wp-content/uploads/sites/460/2018/10/Crossing-the-Quality-Chasm.pdf. (p. 63-64). Last accessed on March 18, 2024.

> health. Such trust involves patient confidence both that those who are responsible for care have the information they need—regardless of where that information was generated—and that those organizations and caregivers will act in patients' best interests and actively seek to advance their health.[32]

Healthcare professionals, like all humans, are fallible. Despite their best efforts, mistakes can occur due to forgetfulness, distraction, or human error. However, these errors continue and even increase in the absence of an error-prevention system. Also, organisational issues, such as inadequate staffing levels, poor workflow processes, or lack of standardised protocols, contribute to errors.

While diagnosing medical conditions can be challenging, and errors in diagnosis are not uncommon, Medication errors, such as prescribing the wrong medication, incorrect dosage, or administration errors, are among the most common types of mistakes in healthcare delivery. And when medication involves biological drugs, errors can indeed be crippling and fatal.

> Errors increase with complexity. Complexity in the medication system arises from several sources; including the extensive knowledge and information that are necessary to correctly prescribe a medication regimen for a particular patient; the intermingling of medications of varying hazards in the pharmacy, during transport, and on the patient care units; and the multiple tasks performed by nurses, of which medication preparation and administration are but a few.

32 Ibid. p. 46.

> Because the burden of harm to patients is great, the cost to society is large, and knowledge of how to prevent the most common kinds of errors is well known, the committee singles out medication safety as a high priority area for all healthcare organizations.[33]

As the next step to the two excellent relations – healthcare delivery happens under a system, and to err is human - the HSS seeks to understand how different healthcare system components interact and how they can be optimised to improve outcomes for patients and populations. Like the aviation industry, the healthcare industry must also operate under a regulatory system of checks and balances ranging from purely technical errors to maintenance related issues, coordination, and interfacing between various systems, and above all human errors.

As we progress into the 21st century, several factors indicate the growing importance of HSS by fostering collaboration, innovation, and a focus on improving health outcomes for individuals and populations alike. Incorporating HSS into healthcare education and training programs ensures that future generations of healthcare professionals are equipped with the knowledge and skills necessary to navigate the complexities of modern healthcare systems. This last and concluding chapter presents six critical areas of HSS - Healthcare Delivery Models, Quality Improvement and Patient Safety, Health Policy, Healthcare Economics, Healthcare Technology, and Population Health.

33 https://nap.nationalacademies.org/download/9728. (p. 183). Last accessed on March 18, 2024.

I now present my observations about the Indian healthcare delivery systems. The idea is not to criticise it because it is what it could be. The idea is to present a wholesome picture to the young doctor, who may sink into despair by being stuck in a particularly stifled situation. Models vary widely due to the country's diverse population, infrastructure, and healthcare needs.

India has a vast public healthcare system that provides healthcare services through government-run facilities such as primary health centres (PHCs), community health centres (CHCs), district hospitals, and tertiary care hospitals. These facilities offer the population subsidised or free healthcare services, particularly in rural and underserved areas. The private healthcare sector in India is also extensive and diverse, ranging from small clinics and nursing homes to large corporate hospitals and speciality centres. Private healthcare providers play a significant role in delivering healthcare services, particularly in urban areas, and often cater to patients seeking better amenities and specialised care. Non-Governmental Organizations (NGOs): Several NGOs operate healthcare facilities and programs across India, especially in rural and marginalised communities. These organisations often focus on providing primary healthcare services, preventive care, maternal and child health services, and health education. With the increasing penetration of mobile phones and internet connectivity, telemedicine and digital health platforms are gaining popularity in India. These platforms enable remote consultations, medical advice, and the delivery of healthcare services, particularly in areas with limited access to healthcare facilities.

The health insurance sector in India is growing rapidly, with various public and private insurance companies offering health insurance plans to individuals and families. Health insurance coverage facilitates access to healthcare services in private hospitals and clinics, covering medical expenses and reducing out-of-pocket expenditures for patients. Launched by the Government of India, Ayushman Bharat is the world's largest government-funded healthcare program. It aims to provide health insurance coverage to over 500 million vulnerable individuals and families, offering cashless access to healthcare services in empanelled public and private hospitals.

Quality improvement and patient safety are critical aspects of healthcare delivery in India, and efforts to enhance both have been gaining momentum in recent years. Accreditation bodies such as the National Accreditation Board for Hospitals & Healthcare Providers (NABH) and the National Accreditation Board for Testing and Calibration Laboratories (NABL) are crucial in promoting quality standards and patient safety in healthcare facilities. Hospitals and laboratories accredited by these bodies adhere to stringent quality and safety protocols.

Many healthcare organisations in India have implemented clinical governance frameworks to ensure accountability, transparency, and continuous improvement in clinical practices. This involves establishing clinical quality committees, conducting regular clinical audits, and implementing evidence-based clinical guidelines. Healthcare facilities increasingly encourage patient feedback and complaints as part of their quality improvement initiatives. Feedback from patients and their families provides valuable insights into areas for improvement and helps identify gaps in service delivery. Adopting health information technology (HIT) solutions such as electronic health records (EHRs), clinical decision support systems, and patient safety software helps improve care coordination, reduce medical errors, and enhance patient safety by ensuring accurate and timely information exchange among healthcare providers.

However, creating a safety culture within healthcare organisations is a work in progress. There is awareness about fostering open communication, reporting adverse events, and learning from errors. Initiatives such as safety huddles, root cause analysis, and safety briefings promote a proactive approach to identifying and addressing patient safety risks. Healthcare professionals across various disciplines receive training on quality improvement methodologies, patient safety principles, and error prevention strategies. Professional organisations and academic institutions offer continuous medical education programs, workshops, and certification courses on patient safety and quality improvement.

Besides, India has a rich tradition of traditional and alternative systems of medicine, such as Ayurveda, Yoga, Naturopathy, Unani, Siddha, and Homeopathy (AYUSH). These systems coexist with modern allopathic medicine, and many people in India seek healthcare services from traditional medicine practitioners for various ailments. It is a massive and deeply entrenched system and has been serving millions of people to pronounced beneficial effects. These healthcare delivery models operate in tandem, often complementing each other to meet the diverse healthcare needs of India's population. However, challenges such as inadequate infrastructure, healthcare workforce shortages, inequitable distribution of healthcare resources, and gaps in quality and accessibility persist and require continuous attention and innovation.

Health policy in India is a multifaceted area of governance encompassing a wide range of initiatives, regulations, and programs aimed at improving the health and well-being of the population. The Government of India is central in formulating and implementing health policies through various ministries and departments, including the Ministry of Health and Family Welfare (MoHFW). National health policies outline the government's vision, priorities, and strategies for addressing healthcare challenges and improving health outcomes. Achieving universal health coverage (UHC) is a cornerstone of India's health policy agenda. Initiatives such as Ayushman Bharat aim to expand access to healthcare services and provide financial protection against catastrophic health expenses for vulnerable populations through health insurance coverage. Strengthening primary healthcare services is a crucial focus of health policy in India. India's health policy framework encourages collaboration between the public and private sectors to address healthcare challenges effectively. PPP models are utilised to improve service delivery, infrastructure development, and healthcare financing, particularly in underserved areas.

Health policy in India includes regulations and standards governing healthcare delivery, medical education, pharmaceuticals, medical devices, and food safety. Regulatory bodies such as the Central Drugs Standard Control Organization (CDSCO) and the Medical Council of India (MCI) oversee quality and safety standards compliance. There are significant social determinants of health, such as poverty, education, sanitation, and access to clean water, as integral components of public health interventions. Despite considerable progress, challenges such as inadequate healthcare infrastructure, healthcare workforce shortages, inequitable access to healthcare services, and persistent health disparities remain. Addressing these challenges requires sustained investment, multisectoral collaboration, community engagement, and evidence-based policy interventions to achieve the health goal for all in India.

Healthcare economics in India is a complex field that involves studying various factors influencing the country's production, consumption, and distribution of healthcare goods and services. India's healthcare expenditure includes public and private spending on healthcare goods and services. Public spending on healthcare is relatively low compared to many other countries, leading to significant out-of-pocket spending by individuals and households, particularly for outpatient care and medications. Healthcare financing mechanisms in India encompass a mix of public, private, and out-of-pocket expenditures. Government-funded health insurance schemes, such as Ayushman Bharat, aim to provide financial protection to vulnerable populations. In contrast, private health insurance and employer-sponsored health plans offer coverage to the urban middle-class and formal sector workers. The private healthcare sector in India is extensive and diverse, ranging from small clinics and nursing homes to large corporate hospitals and speciality centres. Private healthcare providers are significant in delivering healthcare services, particularly in urban areas, and cater to patients seeking better amenities and specialised care.

There is no denying the fact that access to healthcare services in India varies widely across regions, with urban areas generally having better access to healthcare facilities and services compared to rural and remote areas, yet it is also a fact that India is attracting patients from around the world – especially Africa - seeking high-quality healthcare services at relatively lower costs. So while world standards have been achieved in healthcare delivery, they are limited to certain hospitals and available to those who can pay for their treatment. Achieving equity in healthcare access and addressing disparities in healthcare outcomes remain significant challenges.

India faces challenges related to inadequate healthcare infrastructure, including shortages of hospital beds, healthcare professionals, medical equipment, and essential medicines, particularly in rural and underserved areas. Investments in healthcare infrastructure are imperative to meet the growing demand for healthcare services. There is a need for more healthcare professionals, including doctors, nurses, and allied health workers, relative to its population size. Challenges related to maternal and child mortality, infectious diseases, malnutrition, and non-communicable diseases (NCDs) remain dogging, if not unsurmountable.

Adopting electronic health records and digital health record systems improves patient data management, care coordination, and clinical decision-making in healthcare facilities across

India. Health information exchange (HIE) platforms enable the seamless sharing of patient health information among healthcare providers, laboratories, pharmacies, and other stakeholders. HIE promotes interoperability, care coordination, and informed decision-making, ultimately enhancing the quality and efficiency of healthcare delivery. The widespread use of smartphones has led to the proliferation of mobile health applications (mHealth apps) catering to various healthcare needs, such as appointment scheduling, medication reminders, health monitoring, fitness tracking, and teleconsultations. These apps empower users to take control of their health and wellness.

Remote monitoring devices, including wearable sensors, smartwatches, and medical IoT (Internet of Things) devices, enable continuous monitoring of vital signs, chronic conditions, and wellness parameters outside traditional healthcare settings. Remote monitoring enhances preventive care, early detection of health issues, and patient engagement in self-management. Artificial Intelligence (AI) and Machine Learning (ML) technologies are increasingly being integrated into healthcare systems in India to support clinical decision-making, disease diagnosis, risk prediction, and personalised treatment planning. I can see AI-powered tools analysing large volumes of medical data, including imaging scans, genomic information, and patient records, to derive actionable insights and improve healthcare outcomes in premier institutions. Healthcare analytics platforms are deployed, and attempts are being made to identify trends, patterns, and opportunities for quality improvement, cost optimisation, and population health management.

Fintech solutions are transforming healthcare financing and insurance processes, making it easier for individuals to access health insurance coverage, manage healthcare expenses, and make cashless transactions at healthcare facilities. Insurtech platforms streamline insurance claims processing, policy management, and customer engagement. Overall, healthcare technology plays a transformative role in India's healthcare landscape, improving access, affordability, and quality of care while driving innovation and efficiency across the healthcare continuum. Continued investment, collaboration, and regulatory support are essential to harness the full potential of healthcare technology and address the evolving healthcare needs of India's population.

This brings me to the final point of population health, a multifaceted concept encompassing the health outcomes and determinants of the entire population or specific segments. India has a diverse population with variations in age, gender, socioeconomic status, ethnicity, and geography. Demographic factors influence health outcomes and health disparities across different population groups. Social determinants such as education, income, occupation, housing, sanitation, and access to clean water significantly impact population health in India. Addressing social determinants is crucial for improving health equity and reducing health inequalities.

Health behaviours such as diet, physical activity, tobacco use, alcohol consumption, and preventive healthcare practices influence population health outcomes. Addressing unhealthy behaviours and promoting healthy lifestyles through education, awareness campaigns, and policy interventions is essential for improving population health. Environmental factors such as air pollution, water pollution, sanitation, climate change, and occupational hazards impact population health in India. Implementing policies and interventions to mitigate environmental risks and promote environmental sustainability is essential for protecting public health. Addressing the determinants of health and implementing comprehensive, multisectoral strategies are necessary for improving population health outcomes and reducing health inequities across the country.

Medical education and public health have historically operated in separate spheres. The former has traditionally focused on individual patient care, often to the exclusion of a broader public health perspective. However, a growing understanding of the necessity of incorporating public health principles into medical education exists. This prepares better healthcare professionals to address significant health issues impacting communities and populations. Notably, there are active initiatives to bridge this gap, aiming to create a more comprehensive approach to healthcare.

The primary goal of medical education is to train healthcare professionals to provide the best possible care for patients. However, some critiques suggest that the traditional structure of medical education, which often focuses heavily on theoretical knowledge and clinical skills, may sometimes result in a disconnect from the more humanistic aspects of patient care, such as communication, empathy, and patient-centred care. Medical schools must integrate these critical elements into the curriculum to ensure that future healthcare providers are well-rounded and can provide excellent patient care.

I must leave this book in your hands now with my take on what should or could happen in medicine. Predicting the exact state of India's healthcare system by 2030 involves considering various factors, including current trends, ongoing reforms, and emerging challenges. No one can provide a precise forecast, but here is my speculative view of what the healthcare system in India might look like by 2030.

India will make significant strides towards achieving universal health coverage (UHC). Ayushman Bharat and ongoing reforms in public health insurance schemes would contribute to expanding access to healthcare services and providing financial protection to a more significant population segment. The increased adoption of health information technology solutions, electronic health records, telemedicine, and digital health platforms would enhance access to healthcare services, improve care coordination, and improve health outcomes through data-driven decision-making. Healthcare workforce shortages will be met, and skill gaps will be filled by investing in medical education, training, and capacity building.

Innovation in healthcare delivery, technology, and financing models will thrive, driven by increased public-private collaborations, entrepreneurship, and investments in research and development. Innovations like point-of-care, precision medicine, AI-driven diagnostics, and personalised healthcare solutions could revolutionise healthcare delivery. With rising awareness of the importance of preventive healthcare and wellness, India may prioritise initiatives to promote healthy lifestyles, disease prevention, and early detection of health risks. India has the potential to emerge as a global leader in healthcare innovation, research, and healthcare delivery by 2030. Collaborations with international partners, participation in global health initiatives, and contributions to addressing global health challenges could enhance India's stature in the global healthcare landscape.

As we stand on the threshold of incredible breakthroughs and innovations, remember the sacred duty bestowed upon us: the relentless pursuit of healing, progress, and compassion. The baton of medical science has been passed down through generations, a symbol of our collective commitment to the betterment of humanity. Today, as we witness unprecedented strides in healthcare, we must reaffirm our dedication to the noble cause that binds us.

Let us carry this baton with unwavering resolve, knowing that with each step, we bring hope to the afflicted, comfort to the suffering, and light to the darkest corners of despair. But let us remember the weight of this responsibility. The baton should not fall. It carries with it the hopes and dreams of millions, the promise of a healthier, brighter future. In our hands lies the power to transform lives, conquer diseases once thought impossible, and alter the story of human suffering.

So let us march onward, fuelled by the spirit of inquiry, driven by the belief that no challenge is too great, no obstacle too daunting. Let us collaborate, innovate, and persevere, knowing that we are unstoppable. The baton must not fall, for in its journey lies the salvation of countless souls. Let us carry it with pride, purpose, and unwavering determination. For the sake of all those who have come before us, for the sake of all those who will come after us, the baton should not fall. Move forward with courage and conviction.

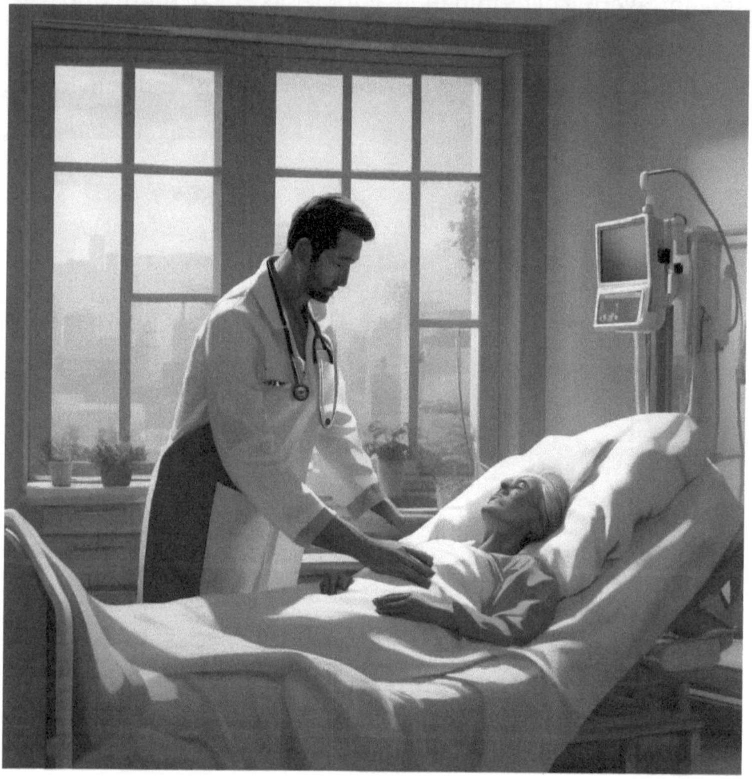

Epilogue

> So do not set a price on yourself. Do not measure out your professional services . . . Do not debase yourself by equating your souls to what they will bring in the market . . . be reckless and spendthrift, pouring out your talent to all to whom it can be of service.[34]
>
> Judge Elbert P. Tuttle

How do I conclude this book? The ten chapters convey the basic theme of a medical doctor's work as part of the legacy of knowledge and service passed on by successive generations in the hands of younger ones. I have chosen the words of American Judge Elbert P. Tuttle (1897-1996), who said that 'to be professional' was the most significant achievement of a human life. Every child grows up learning every day from people around him – mainly family and community. Then comes school and, eventually, higher education. But with no character build-up, the career collapses like a house built on a weak foundation.

---

34 https://www.ca11.uscourts.gov/remembering-judge-elbert-p-tuttle. Last accessed on July 23, 2024.

A character is typically defined by a combination of traits, qualities, and characteristics that shape who they are. These aspects can include their personality, beliefs, values, motivations, strengths, weaknesses, and how they interact with others. An important aspect of character development is growth and change over time, as characters face challenges, make decisions, and experience different situations that influence their development. Well-rounded characters often have depth, complexity, and a sense of authenticity, allowing others to connect with and relate to them.

The practice of medicine has indeed been a longstanding tradition that dates back centuries. While medicine has seen remarkable advancements in technology and treatments, many core principles of medicine, such as compassion, empathy, dedication to healing, and the importance of patient care, have remained timeless. The traditions of medicine continue to evolve, incorporating new scientific discoveries and technologies while upholding the fundamental values that have guided healthcare professionals for generations.

The secret of success in medicine is caring for ' the person' in every patient, not merely his disease or ailment. Teaching and mentoring the students and junior colleagues and sharing one's successes. Be it recognition and fame or material gains, the team is part of this generous and empathetic approach with them. The team is, after all, an extended family of the physician. Today, this mentoring and sharing need to be broadly inclusive, involving the more comprehensive healthcare delivery system, which also becomes part of this large extended family.

We must be humble enough to continue to be students and make all this possible, which may never be attainable in one's lifetime. This is an unfinished and infinite journey of medicine. This incredible journey and unending game may never be achieved in one's lifetime. Our children and grandchildren carry forward our genomic structures, but our intellectual, academic, and character strengths and professional legacy are carried forward, on and on, by our students, colleagues, and friends. Some may leave, but others join.

We must be humble enough to continue to be students and make [illegible]

Acknowledgements

I have spent over two decades with Dr B. Soma Raju. I met him as a patient in 1987 while working at the Defence Research & Development Laboratory in Hyderabad. Our meeting turned into a friendship, which led to the creation of Civilian Spinoffs of Defence Technology to make expensive medical devices and materials affordable and accessible to patients for most who need them but are cost-prohibitive.

In 1997, I started working full-time with Dr Raju. We tried many things through Care Foundation and Care Hospitals; some succeeded, and many failed. But what truly transformed me in that process was the profound impact of Dr Raju's substantial personal library, where he collected rare books. I have read many of them over the years. This book has been churned out of those books as an attempt to share with young doctors a "sip of the nectar."

Medicine is a hallowed profession, and I find myself a rare species to have entered its inner ring without being a doctor. Dr M. Srinivas, Director, AIIMS, has written the Foreword, which has sanctified this endeavour. He is a true Karma Yogi, I ever met.

Writing this book has been a very satisfying experience, made possible by the collaboration of many talented individuals. I was assisted by Dr Sunkavalli Chinnababu, a Surgical Oncologist and and founder-CEO of Grace Cancer Foundation; Dr Vipin Das, an Ophthalmologist-researcher; the Care Foundation team headed by Mr S.G. Prasad, and the Sakal Publications editorial team under Mr Ashutosh Ramgir's leadership.

Arun Tiwari

Index

AIIMS, The All India Institutes of Medical Sciences, New Delhi, 14, 101
AYUSH, Ayurveda, Yoga, Naturopathy, Unani, Siddha, and Homeopathy systems, 180
CIHS, Care Institute of Health Sciences, Hyderabad, 95
EMRI, Emergency Management and Research Institute, Hyderabad, 95
IMA, Indian Medical Association, 119
IMTECH, Institute of Microbial Technology, Chandigarh, 109
IPPNW, International Physicians for the Prevention of Nuclear War, Geneva, 123
IOM, the Institute of Medicine in the U.S., 174
NABH, National Accreditation Board for Hospitals and Healthcare Providers in India, 16, 179
NEET, National Eligibility cum Entrance Test in India, 16
NIAID, National Institute of Allergy and Infectious Diseases in U.S., 69
NIMS, Nizam's Institute of Medical Sciences, Hyderabad, 9
NMC, National Medical Commission of India, 16
PGI, Postgraduate Institute of Medical Education and Research, Chandigarh, 9, 15, 56
WHO, World Health Organization, 26

A

Aequanimitas, book, 12, 37, 72
Albert Einstein, Physicist, Nobel Laurette, 75,
Alexis Carrel, Dr., Nobel Laurette
Man, The Unknown, book, 71

Amartya Sen, Indian Economist, Nobel Laurette, 112
American Medical Association Journal, JAMA, 64
Anganwadi workers, 105
Anthony Fauci, American physician-scientist, 69
Artificial intelligence (AI), 13, 51, 68, 110, 120, 133, 184
Ayurveda, 13, 180

B

Bernard Lown, Lithuanian-American cardiologist and inventor, 123
British Medical Association, 26

C

COVID-19, 68, 69, 116
Care Foundation
  Hospitals, 9
  Institute of Health Sciences, 95
Competency-based medical education (CBME), 17
CRISPR–Cas9, Gene editing technology, 68, 109

D

David Sackett, American-Canadian physician, 62
  Evidence-based medicine, 63
Dennis Kasper, American microbiologist and immunologist, 69

E

Eddy, David M., American physician, mathematician, and healthcare analyst, 173
Elbert P. Tuttle, American judge, 191
Evidence-based medicine (EBM)
  Levels of evidence, 12, 60, 62, 64, 68

G

Gulapalli Nageswara Rao, Ophthalmologist, 133
Guntaka, Ramareddy V, Biotechnology scientist, 109
Guntur Medical College, 12, 37, 55
Guthrie, Charles C., American physiologist, 74

H

Harvey Cushing, American neurosurgeon and pathologist, 74
Healthcare economics, 173, 177, 182
Health Systems Science, 32, 173

Henry Dakin, English chemist, 80
Hippocrates, ancient Greek philosopher, 11, 23, 65, 109, 114, 126, 141
  Corpus, 23
  Oath, 24
  Revised Oath, 28

I
Immune checkpoint inhibitors, 69

J
Jameson, Larry J., American physician-scientist, 69
John Brown, Scottish physician, 26, 27
Joseph Loscalzo, Professor of Medicine, Harvard Medical School, 69
Johns Hopkins School of Medicine, 37, 75
Journal of Medical Internet Research, 32

K
Kalam, A.P.J., President of India, 9, 13, 84, 85, 94
  Kalam-Raju Stent, 84, 197
  Wings of Fire, book, 9
Karl Landsteiner, Austrian American biologist, Nobel Laurette, 75

L
Lois DeBakey, Lebanese-American scientific communicator, 157, 158
Longo, Dan L, Professor of Medicine at Harvard Medical School, 69
Louis Lasagna, American Physician, 28
LV Prasad Eye Institute, 133

M
Manning, Phil R., American doctor, 157
  Society for Academic Continuing Medical Education
Matthew Effect, 65

O
Osmania Medical College 9
Outcomes Management (OM), 63

P
Pellegrino, Edmund Daniel, American bioethicist and academic, 107
Physician Assistants, 93, 94, 95, 104, 105
Prasad, B.N, Orthopaedic Surgeon, 85
  Floor Reaction Orthosis, 85

R

Raju, G.S., Industrialist, 14
Rama Raju, G., Industrialist, 108
Rudolph Matas, American Surgeon, 75

S

Seamus O'Mahony, Irish medical doctor and author, 143
Socially Assistive Robots (SARs), 136
Stead, Eugene A., American physician, medical educator, 89
Stephen Hauser, American Neurologist, 69

T

Tinsley Harrison, American cardilogist, 7, 55, 123
Principles of Internal Medicine, book, 55, 59, 69

V

von Schelling, German philosopher, 27

W

White, Paul D., American cardiologist, 159, 160
William Halstead, American surgeon, 75
William Harvey, 11
William Osler, American medical doctor, educator, 7, 37, 55, 65, 75, 123
William Welch, American physician and pathologist, 75